AFRICA

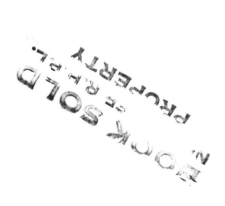

A PRACTICAL GUIDE
FOR GLOBAL HEALTH
WORKERS

AFRICA

LAUREL A. SPIELBERG

LISA V. ADAMS

EDITORS

DARTMOUTH

COLLEGE PRESS

HANOVER, NEW HAMPSHIRE

DARTMOUTH COLLEGE PRESS

Published by University Press of New England

www.upne.com

© 2011 Trustees of Dartmouth College

All rights reserved

Manufactured in the United States of America

Designed by Eric M. Brooks

Typeset in Fresco and Fresco Sans

by Passumpsic Publishing

University Press of New England is a member of the
Green Press Initiative. The paper used in this book meets
their minimum requirement for recycled paper.

For permission to reproduce any of the material in this
book, contact Permissions, University Press of New England,
One Court Street, Suite 250, Lebanon NH 03766; or visit
www.upne.com

Library of Congress Cataloging-in-Publication Data
appear on the last printed page of this book.

5 4 3 2 1

**WE DEDICATE THIS BOOK
TO OUR CHILDREN**

*The privilege of being the parent of Lucas and
Lea Adams-Blackmore has made me a better doctor,
educator, and person. Their enthusiasm for life constantly
buoys me — my wish that every child may feel the hope
and excitement I see in their eyes is what motivates
me every day.*

LVA

*David and Jeff Spielberg, who are engaged on their
own paths to bettering the world, will recognize their
individual contributions to ideas in this book.
They inspire me daily.*

LAS

CONTENTS

There are a multitude of opportunities to work in Africa on health or humanitarian aid projects sponsored by non-profit organizations, religious organizations, schools, and universities. These experiences can be broadening and life changing, and can help prepare you for a career of service with a global perspective.

We recognized, however, that there is little information for potential volunteers and travelers that focuses on health, or provides a context for understanding what you will find when you arrive at your African destination. What we have commonly heard when our students return from experiences abroad is: "It would have helped if I had known . . ." or "I wish I had been better prepared for what I was going to see." This book attempts to address some of the gaps.

In the first chapter, the book gives an overview of humanitarianism and the concepts underlying global health. The chapter also provides a specific focus on the context of health in Africa, as background for traveling there to do global health work. The second chapter provides a wide range of practical tips for planning your trip and for engaging successfully in the work you aim to do in Africa. The following seven chapters on individual countries — and, in one case, on a region — provide a socio-cultural, political, legal, health system, and disease epidemiology context for readers. The chapter authors share their own experiences with health initiatives and research projects undertaken in specific African countries. The book's final chapter provides useful advice for making the most of your work experience in Africa and re-adjusting when you return home. The book's glossary provides definitions of terms, agencies and diseases you are likely to encounter.

The book does not attempt to cover all global health aspects of the African continent. Rather, we have chosen seven representative countries or regions. They vary in size from tiny to large, and in population from sparsely to the most densely populated. They also represent a fair portion of the continent's geography, from North Africa (Morocco, Algeria and Tunisia), East Africa (Uganda and United Republic of Tanzania), Central Africa (Rwanda), West Africa (Ghana), and Southern Africa (Botswana and South Africa).

Numerous authors contributed to this book. Each author has had many years of practical experience in the African country he or she discusses, and shares information about Africa from their individual perspective and experience as actors and collaborators on the ground, developing and running health and human rights projects and programs. Most of the authors we invited to contribute to the book are faculty members at U.S.-based universities or medical institutions. All are actively involved in an ongoing way in the country they write about. Immediately, many authors invited one or more African colleagues to write the chapter with them. This shared authorship gives an additional perspective and depth to the material they present. The resulting pictures of each country and its challenges are surprisingly candid and forceful. Yet you will detect in each chapter the authors' love of the country and its people, and their enthusiasm for the work they are doing there.

Having different authors for each country chapter has resulted in a portrait of each country that is intimate and knowledgeable. At the same time, it has resulted in a variety of styles and choices in what each chapter covers, largely based on the expertise, orientation, and experiences of the respective authors, which are highlighted in their brief biographies in the Contributors section at the end of the book.

Each country chapter focuses on different aspects of health, service delivery, or human rights. Some issues are discussed in nearly every chapter, such as HIV/AIDS, tuberculosis and malaria, diseases that are very prevalent in many African countries. Many of the authors came to their work with specific expertise in infectious diseases, and they bring this perspective to the African experiences they share here. Despite these similarities, not every chapter covers every health topic or covers the same topic in the same way. Readers who want to gain a varied perspective can read about a topic in several chapters by looking up the topic in the book's index. Doing so will give you a broader perspective on a topic than reading a single chapter. For instance, the South African government's approach to HIV/AIDS contrasted sharply with the approach taken by the government of Botswana in the early years of the epidemic. Reading about HIV/AIDS in both country chapters offers a sharp contrast and a compelling lesson in what can be achieved when science underpins decision-making, and drives a government to act promptly.

It is also important to remember that although chapter authors focus attention on a problem within a single country, in fact, the problem may be ubiquitous throughout Africa: the childhood mortality and malnutrition described in the Rwanda and Tanzania chapters, the high rates of maternal mortality and septic abortion described in the Maghreb chapter, and the Ghana chapter's highlighting of the high toll of traffic accidents and lack of emergency medical capacity to address these needs are good examples. These are problems throughout most of Africa.

Besides focusing on a specific country and its significant health or human rights issues, each chapter offers something for all readers—a broader perspective on some topic that will be of interest no matter where you are going in Africa. A highlight of the Botswana chapter, for instance, is its introduction to some outstanding and memorable African literature—an enjoyable way to prepare for travels abroad. The Ghana chapter gives special consideration to African cultural beliefs and their influence on health behaviors and use of health care. The Maghreb chapter provides a unique focus on women's rights in three countries in northwest Africa. The chapter continually highlights connections between women's rights, women's health and reproductive outcomes, and the health of families. The authors of the Rwanda chapter share the wrenching impact of a devastating event in the country's history, the 1994 genocide, and the country's efforts to rebuild, overcome, and emerge a better nation. Rwanda has the highest burden of orphans in Africa, and the authors provide a moving glimpse into the world of orphans, vulnerable children and child-headed households. The South African chapter illustrates the persistence of history in its moving descriptions of the legacy of apartheid in the country today. The chapter on Tanzania pays particular attention to the many international organizations working in Africa, and underscores the inter-relatedness and partnership building that are so essential in global health work. The Uganda chapter introduces you to zoonotic diseases and their potential impact on both human and animal health in a largely pastoral country.

We hope you will see this book as more than a travel guide to specific countries. Reading about multiple countries will allow you to compare and contrast them, giving you a perspective from which to view any country. At the end of each chapter, we provide facts and figures that will tell you about various aspects of the country's demography, sociology, economics, environment and health. These indicators can be viewed as tools to help you approach thinking about a country — even your own country of origin — in terms of the interweaving of human rights, health, and health care. All the data and references in this book were up to date at the time the book went to press. However, references — and particularly internet sources — change quickly these days. We encourage you to seek updated resources if those provided here are no longer current or available.

Collectively, these chapters emphasize the challenges of improving health in the face of poverty, lack of education, inadequate infrastructure, strained resources, and inequitable distribution of opportunities. The book makes it clear that global health is inextricably interwoven with politics, economics and policy.

We hope you will read all the chapters for a broad and rich perspective.

ACKNOWLEDGMENTS

The many students we have counseled before their travels to Africa, throughout their endeavors, and after their return provided the motivation for this book. They, above all, have inspired us with their curiosity, ability to translate ideas into action, and determination to make the world a better place. We have learned from their experiences, and hope that we have articulated their lessons into information others can readily use.

We are grateful to the many authors who contributed their knowledge and experiences to so thoughtfully describe the countries profiled in this book. All unselfishly shared their enthusiasm, dedication, expertise, and love of the country they wrote about.

In addition, several authors contributed tips and advice that are highly relevant for all travelers to Africa, and this information has been incorporated into the book's second chapter. For their wisdom and forethought in this regard, we particularly thank Joyce A. Sackey, Nameeta M. Dookeran, Stella Safo, and Elizabeth Talbot. Stephanie Willman Bordat and Saida Kouzzi, the authors of the Maghreb chapter, provided critical and sensitive insights into working in a foreign culture. Their tips for helping readers understand cultural differences and develop positive relationships will help anyone working abroad to be more effective.

Our fondest thanks go to Ambassador Kenneth S. Yalowitz, director of the Dickey Center for International Understanding at Dartmouth College, who brought us together as an editorial team, and provided the ongoing encouragement to ensure that we completed this project.

Dr. Phyllis Deutsch, editor in chief of the University Press of New England, recognized at an early stage the potential usefulness of this book, and bolstered us with her enthusiasm for the project. She has provided wise advice throughout the process.

We were fortunate to receive valuable input from several reviewers. Dana C. Grossman, Cynthia Haq, Heather Lukolyo, Stuart M. MacLeod, and Peter Mogielnicki, provided critical and thoughtful insights that improved this book.

Our spouses, Lars Blackmore and Stephen P. Spielberg, have been ever-present boosters and supporters of this project.

Lars is the anchor of our family and household, artfully handling the practical details while providing stability to our otherwise hectic lives. His love and support help me feel grounded wherever my international work takes me and have allowed me to pursue my career with passion. LVA

Stephen Spielberg has made my life an adventure. I am inspired by his vision that allows him to move with ease between an individualized focus on each child and his efforts for children's health globally. LAS

AFRICA

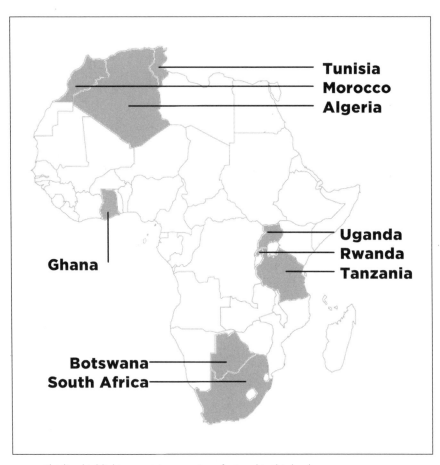

Tunisia
Morocco
Algeria

Ghana

Uganda
Rwanda
Tanzania

Botswana
South Africa

Shading highlights countries or regions featured in this book

1

LISA V. ADAMS

LAUREL A. SPIELBERG

CLAIRE WAGNER

INTRODUCTION

HUMANITARIANISM, GLOBAL HEALTH, AND UNDERSTANDING THE AFRICAN CONTEXT

Understanding Humanitarianism

Humanitarianism is a manifestation of human life and interaction. Simply put, humanitarianism is concern for human welfare. It can be demonstrated through philanthropy and through action. Concern for others is grounded in the view that all human beings deserve respect and dignity, regardless of their condition or situation in life. The right to life with dignity is proclaimed in both the Universal Declaration of Human Rights and the International Covenant on Civil and Political Rights: "All human beings are born free and equal in dignity and human rights."[1] The aim of humanitarian action is to advance the well-being of humanity, provide assistance where requested, save lives, and alleviate human suffering, without regard for ethnicity, nationalism, religion, ancestry, or political viewpoint.

Albert Schweitzer, philosopher, theologian, and physician, is often thought of as a notable example of a humanitarian. In 1913, he founded a hospital at Lambarene in French Equatorial Africa, France's colonies in Middle Africa (which are now the countries of Gabon, Republic of the Congo, Central African Republic, and Chad). The hospital he established

1

continues today, offering medical, surgical, obstetric, pediatric, and dental care, and has a malaria research unit. Modeled on Schweitzer's lifelong humanitarian activities, the U.S. Schweitzer Fellowship program provides opportunities in community service for graduate students in health-related professions. The program's aim is to train what it calls "leaders in service," with the skills to address unmet health needs in communities.[2]

Humanitarian efforts should be undertaken without expectation of reward. However, a well-known symbol of humanitarian efforts, the Nobel Peace Prize, recognizes exemplary efforts and activities that have impacted human conditions in the world. The Nobel Committee regards humanitarian efforts as a key element in promoting peace by improving lives and reducing suffering, narrowing the gaps between rich and poor countries, and strengthening human rights. Over the years, the Peace Prizes have recognized both individuals and organizations for such humanitarian efforts as providing assistance for victims of war and disaster (for instance, the International Committee of the Red Cross in 1917, 1944, and 1963; and the United Nations (UN) High Commissioner for Refugees in 1954 and 1981), promoting pacifism and humanitarianism (the British and American Friends Service Committees in 1947, Albert Schweitzer in 1952, and Mother Theresa in 1979), increasing the world's food supply (Norman Borlaug in 1970), working for the rights and welfare of children (UNICEF in 1965), providing medical aid and supporting human rights (Médecins sans Frontières/Doctors without Borders in 1999), and promoting economic and social development in order to eliminate poverty (Muhammad Yunus and the Grameen Bank in 2006).[3] Awards such as these recognize both global responsibility and the important role of humanitarianism in addressing the world's problems.

Clearly, humanitarian action has a very broad scope and can be directed at many issues that affect the human condition. Humanitarian action is also guided by a long history of legislation intentionally aimed at improving conditions for people, often called social legislation. This type of legislation is a society's way of protecting human welfare, and acknowledging the rights and special needs of its citizens. Examples include laws that address the rights, welfare, and protection of workers, or provide for special groups like children, the unemployed, or those who are elderly, ill, injured, disabled, or poor.[4] Social legislation differs from country to country. The traveler to Africa should be particularly alert to the existence or absence of legislated protections for groups and individuals within a country.

Numerous international treaties and declarations have also helped shape humanitarian efforts and international assistance in the spheres of health, development, economics, food production, disasters and emergencies, and human rights.

Humanitarianism is often the driving force behind emergency responses to crises such as war, famine, displacement, disease outbreaks, or natural disasters. The emphasis of emergency response, sometimes called humanitarian response, is on saving lives and alleviating human suffering. Humanitarian response to disasters in African countries goes back at least as far as the 1970 relief efforts in Biafra. Subsequent famines in the mid-1980s in several African countries, genocide in Rwanda in 1994, and the current situation in the Darfur region of western Sudan have all called attention to the extreme poverty in some areas of Africa, and to the humanitarian crises that result from conflict, hunger, drought, population migration, and refugee status. Several chapters in this book discuss aspects of humanitarian crises: the impacts of genocide (Rwanda); the stresses resulting from population migration (Rwanda, Algeria); problems of families of those who have 'disappeared' (Algeria); orphaned populations (Rwanda, Tanzania); and the impact of the alarming spread of disease (HIV/AIDS and tuberculosis, or TB, in Botswana, Rwanda, South Africa, Tanzania, Uganda).

Core Principles of Humanitarian Efforts

A widely recognized set of principles guide humanitarian activity. These principles evolved from the emergency response activities of organizations such as the International Federation of Red Cross/Red Crescent, the work of nongovernmental organizations (NGOS; see the glossary), and the experience of governmental agencies in providing economic and development assistance to other countries.[5] Today, the following principles guide assistance and humanitarian work throughout the world.

- The most fundamental principle is *humanity*, or respect for human dignity. It means that all people should be treated humanely in all circumstances. Humanitarian efforts should be directed at saving lives and alleviating suffering, while ensuring respect for the individual.

- A second principle is the concept of a *humanitarian imperative*, or the idea that everyone has a right to provide and to receive humanitarian assistance. This principle speaks to the obligation of the international community "to provide humanitarian assistance wherever it is needed."[6]

- In addition, humanitarian action should be based on *impartiality*. That is, it should be need-based and not biased in favor of or against any nationality, race, religion, class or political viewpoints. Impartiality, then, is the opposite of discrimination. It suggests that humanitarian action should give priority to the most urgent cases or situations, no matter where they occur or who they affect.

- Organizations and individuals engaged in humanitarian action should be *neutral*, and not take sides in hostilities or engage in controversies that are political, racial, religious, or ideological. Neutrality means that humanitarian aid should be provided in a way that is impartial and independent.[7]

- The principle of *independence* refers to the ability of providers of humanitarian assistance to maintain autonomy, while still respecting the laws of the country in which the assistance or services are being provided. Humanitarian agencies should be able carry out their policies, independent of the actions and policies of governments. This is often difficult for NGOs that may depend, at least in part, on governments for some of their funding.

- Agencies of the United Nations, the International Federation of Red Cross and Red Crescent Societies, and NGOs that adhere to the Red Cross/NGO Code of Conduct, agree *not to engage in proselytism* — that is, not to use their humanitarian activities to promote political or religious beliefs. To do so could be viewed as exploiting people who are vulnerable. If an agency is perceived as trying to spread a religious faith that is different from local religious beliefs, its humanitarian activities may meet with hostility or resistance.

Additional principles have evolved from countries' and agencies' experiences with development assistance. These are focused on the cultural context and resource capacity of countries receiving the assistance, and include:

- Agencies and individuals should *operate with respect to culture and custom*.

- Humanitarian response should *use local resources and capacities as much as possible.*
- The *beneficiaries should be encouraged to participate* in the humanitarian activity.
- Emergency response should strive to *reduce future vulnerabilities.*
- Agencies should be *accountable to both donors and beneficiaries.*
- Agencies should *portray victims as dignified human beings, not hopeless objects* of external assistance.

Additionally, from a global health perspective, seeking *consent and involvement of the community and individuals being assisted is critical* to their participation and to successful outcomes.

Ensuring adherence to humanitarian principles is undoubtedly difficult. Many agencies monitor themselves and examine issues of compliance internally. The Steering Committee for Humanitarian Response, an alliance of major international humanitarian organizations, carries out peer review among its member agencies to assess their adherence to humanitarian principles.

Globalism and Global Health

Globalism, as used in this book, refers to the reality of being interconnected around the world. The issues talked about in this book, such as disease, nutritional status, access to health care, and literacy are universal. However, because of political, social, and economic forces, they result in differences between people and between countries in economic wellbeing, education, health and environment. Today, the connections between economics, health, and foreign policy are becoming increasingly tighter. Often the boundaries between domestic and foreign issues blur, particularly when it comes to health. Global health is concerned with health issues and the health of populations, without traditional regard for national boundaries. Sometimes the focus of concern is a disease that can spread from country to country. Sometimes the focus is on health issues that are of such magnitude that they can have global economic and political impact. The primary aims of global health are to improve population health, reduce the existing disparities in health between population groups, and protect populations from health threats. A characteristic of global health is that its activities are best carried out in ways that are collaborative and cooperative, and involve multiple interested parties and partners, often from a variety of disciplines.

To understand global health, you need only to think about some headline issues of the last two decades. HIV/AIDS, recognized first in small groups of gay men and then intravenous drug users in California and New York in 1981, has become a pandemic. Severe Acute Respiratory Syndrome (SARS) began in China and Hong Kong, then spread to Canada, highlighting the need for global coordination in order to control the spread of an infectious disease. Preparedness and prevention efforts against bioterrorism have become the focus of global security and health initiatives since the events of 9/11 (11 September 2001) in the United States. When the World Health Organization declared outbreaks of the H1N1 (initially called swine flu) influenza virus a pandemic in June 2009, there were cases in more than seventy countries. In August 2010, WHO declared an end to the H1N1 pandemic, but warned that the virus discovered in 2009 will likely continue to circulate globally for years to come, like a regular seasonal influenza virus.[8]

Understanding the African Context

Anyone traveling to Africa to do global health or humanitarian aid work needs to understand the socio-cultural, political, economic, and historical context of the region. You will need to view Africa and health through a variety of lenses, remembering that each country is diverse in population and culture. In the following section, we provide an overview of specific historical phenomena and socio-cultural factors in Africa's past that influence health, as an introduction to the African context. Because the health system in most African countries differs markedly from that in the United States, we also provide an overview of the typical healthcare delivery system in Africa. By necessity, the introduction to African history provided here is extremely brief. While we provide a general overview, later chapters deal in far greater depth with the history, healthcare system, and leading health issues in particular countries, and the readings recommended at the end of many chapters are excellent additional resources.

To understand Africa today, it's important to understand the continent's history. Enormously diverse, Africa comprises fifty-four countries. It is the second largest continent geographically and the second most populous (after Asia). This book highlights six African countries and one region, a small sampling of the continent's diversity. Our very brief overview of Africa's history emphasizes historical events, and social and cultural trends that have created a lasting legacy on the people of Africa, and their current circumstances. The trans-Atlantic slave trade, the colonial and postcolonial eras, countries' struggles for independence, and, more recently, the imposition of structural economic reforms have had profound effects on health, economics, and human rights in Africa.

A Brief Historical Overview

Early African history suggests that people lived in tribal groupings that settled and adapted their lifestyles to the geographic and physical environment. They were farmers in fertile river valleys that supported agriculture; hunters and gatherers in savannas; shepherds and herdsmen on wooded and grassy ranges; and developed towns in communities along the coasts. Coastal communities had lucrative trading relationships with seafaring and trade route travelers from Mediterranean, Asian, and eventually European countries. Some of history's most remarkable and cultured civilizations formed in Africa, including Alexandria, Cairo, and Carthage.

The Slave Trade

Colonization of the Americas, mostly by Spain and Portugal, and the growth of plantation-style agriculture were seen as a way to meet the increasing European demand for food, sugar, and spices. Plantation-style agriculture drove a demand for inexpensive labor, which the colonies sought to fill with African slaves. Beginning about 1510, Africans were forcibly removed from their homes and communities, sold as slaves to meet American (and sometimes European) demands for laborers, and transported from the west coast of Africa across the Atlantic to the New World. Many African merchants participated in the trade by capturing other Africans and selling them to Europeans in exchange for manufactured goods. African merchants often did not know where the captured Africans were going or how they would be treated. The European demand for sugar and agricultural goods from French, English, and Dutch West Indian plantations caused the trans-Atlantic slave trade to grow rapidly in the seventeenth century, making slaves Africa's chief export. Approximately 275,000 Africans had been shipped overseas by 1600, an additional 1.3 million during the seventeenth century, over 6 million more during the eighteenth century, and another 1.9 million in the nineteenth century.[9] The English, French, and Portuguese dominated the slave trade, and by the end of the eighteenth century, nearly half of all slaves transported to America came on British ships. As the major embarkation area, the West African coast from the Gold Coast (now Ghana) to the Niger River delta (now in Nigeria) became known as the Slave Coast.[10]

The slave trade appears to have had different effects on different regions of Africa. Some Western African settlements may have benefited economically from the trade. In Eastern Africa where populations were relatively sparse and subsistence meager, communities suffered from the loss of young and healthy people, those most desired by slave traders. This forced African diaspora was a devastating loss of human capital for the continent; it caused the populations of many African nations to stagnate or decline. Above all, the dehumanizing impact of being a salable commodity cast a long shadow of inequity on the people of Africa.

While slavery had been a conventional practice long before, the unmistakable human injustice of the trans-Atlantic slave trade played a part in the fragmentation of many ancient African empires, and destroyed or disrupted the continent's economies. For instance, Timbuktu, a city in the ancient empire of Mali, is believed to have once been the intellectual and financial center of Africa. With its University of Sankore, it became a world renowned center of scholarship, culture and wealth. The slave trade was almost surely a contributing factor to the economic decline of such African cultures.

The Anti-Slave Trade Movement

In 1771, activists in Europe began to publicly denounce the slave trade. Under growing abolitionist pressure, the English Parliament made slave trading illegal for Britons in 1807. The imposition of heavy penalties for slave trading essentially caused an end to the trade by Britain in 1811. By about 1842, transportation of slaves across the Atlantic was considered an illegal activity in nearly all American and European countries. However, the world's demands for cotton and sugar kept up a defiant slave market in the United States, Brazil, and Cuba. The slave trade to the United States ended with the 1865 victory of the north in the U.S. civil war. The legacy of economic dependence on the slave trade, and population stagnation in many regions of the African continent helped make it possible for European nations to pursue further economic opportunities in Africa through colonial rule during the nineteenth and twentieth centuries.

European Exploration and Colonization of Africa
The motivation behind Europeans' exploration of Africa in the eighteenth and nineteenth centuries was a combination of curiosity, scientific inquiry, missionary efforts, and philanthropic desire to bring progress—as the Europeans defined it—to Africa and its inhabitants. Undoubtedly, while Christianity and some desire to promote commerce were primary drivers of European interest in Africa, the dominating view was one of laissez-faire politics, assuming that contact with Europe and the desire to trade and interchange would stimulate African development.

Beginning in the mid-1800s, France, Britain, Belgium, Spain, Italy, the Netherlands, Germany, and Portugal expanded their rule and influence to different parts of Africa. Colonial rule affected nearly all institutions, politics, and social settings—including government structures, growth and control of certain industries, health practices, and education systems. By the beginning of the twentieth century, European governments were claiming sovereignty over all but six of the roughly forty political units into which the African continent had been divided by European missionaries and exploration. The European countries' scramble to lay claim to African territory may have been due more to their competition with each other in Europe than to a desire to develop colonies and enrich themselves. European colonizers largely ignored their African colonies in the early part of the twentieth century. The overall aim was for African colonies to be largely self-supporting, minimizing the need for aid from the European power. In large part, colonial powers focused on extracting resources from Africa: rubber, ivory, and the mining of ores and gemstones became the most developed economies. Missionaries, rather than colonial governments, became the main educators of African populations in most countries.

The legacies of colonialism differ from country to country. It is helpful to research the particular colonial history and legacy of the region where you are planning to work. At the conclusion of most chapters in this book, the authors have provided relevant references, including information on the country's colonial history and independence.

Independence

The only African countries that remained fully independent throughout the twentieth century were Ethiopia and Liberia; all the rest of Africa experienced varying degrees of occupation, administration, and colonization by European powers. The impetus for independence among African nations gained momentum during World War II, when African nationals of many countries fought in the armies of their European colonizers, well aware of the irony that they fought for freedom and independence in Europe, while their own countries lacked independence. Africa's transition from colonies to independent nations began in 1951 with the independence of Libya from Italy, followed in 1956 by the independence of Morocco and Tunisia from France. The majority of African countries gained their independence during the 1960s, most through peaceful transitions. Each African country has had its own unique path to sovereign status—sometimes troubled by instability, violence, and dictatorship over the ensuing years. In each country chapter in this book, you will find a brief synopsis of the country's history and path to independence.

International Influences and Important Social Concepts

International influences have played a key role in the economic and social development of African nations. In the 1980s, during the era of Ronald Reagan and Margaret Thatcher, the World Bank and the International Monetary Fund imposed a set of so-called structural adjustment programs (see the glossary) on the economies of African countries that sought financial aid. Developing countries that pledged their compliance with certain strict regulations received loans. These regulations emphasized privatization of various public goods, such as natural resources; reduction in social expenditures, such as those for healthcare and education; liberalization of trade to encourage global market competition and economic stimulation; devaluation of currencies; elimination of price controls and subsidies; improvement of governance; and resource extraction. While these policies made changes in the economies of African countries, it is debated whether their impact has helped or harmed developing nations. In regard to health, the structural adjustment programs affected both the supply of health services (by insisting on cuts in health spending) and the demand for health services (by reducing household incomes, thus leaving people with less money for health care). With the ensuing interconnectedness of the global economy, what has resulted are complex and varied economic systems in Africa.

In the moving film *Bamako*, a tribunal hears testimony about the insurmountable debts of African countries incurred in borrowing money, the failure of structural adjustment, the erosion of infrastructure, and the despair that results. A lawyer for the people suggests that appropriate reparations would be "community service for all humanity for eternity."[11] As seen in this film, concerns remain about the economic and socio-cultural legacies of the structural adjustment programs in developing nations.

Typically, we think that health outcomes in any society are largely defined by the society's financial commitments to infrastructure, public health, education, literacy, and sanitation. In many African nations today, the link between poverty and decreased access to health and educational resources is undeniable. Paul Farmer, a physician and medical anthropologist, uses the term "structural violence" to denote the relationship between poverty and health outcomes.[12] The term signifies the impact of structural barriers that inhibit individuals from fulfilling their basic needs such as health and education. Often intangible, these barriers include the historical, political, economic, ecological, geographic, social, and cultural conditions that reduce an individual's freedom in seeking health care and education. The individual is not at fault; rather, social forces, historical processes, and their resulting legacies constrain the individual. Farmer writes: "Structural violence is visited upon all those whose social status denies them access to the fruits of scientific and social progress."[13]

Health in African Contexts

There are vast differences in how people interpret, cope with, and find solutions for various health risks and problems. These differences are key to understanding how, in turn, people interpret issues of health, illness, and well-being. Social and familial networks are often critical in people's choices about where and from whom to seek guidance on health issues and receive health care. Global health workers should be open to the diversity of health practices in Africa and should understand that biomedical practice, as we know it, is not always the norm. Traditional healers are common in many African societies. Studies have shown that approximately 80 percent of people living with AIDS in Africa consult traditional healers, often in conjunction with conventional antiretroviral therapy (ART; see the glossary).[14] Although many traditional healers operate outside of institutional settings, some African medical universities have schools or departments of complementary and traditional medicine, recognizing and supporting the role of traditional healers in health care.[15]

In any part of the world, health issues should be understood not only from a medical viewpoint, but with an understanding of other contributing factors such as education, living conditions, gender issues, and religious and ethnic acceptance. In the chapters that follow, the authors discuss health topics such as HIV/AIDS and reproductive health from both a socio-cultural and a biomedical perspective. Like other parts of the world, many African societies stigmatize those infected with HIV/AIDS, ostracizing them because their disease is considered disgraceful. Sexual relations are inherently personal and generally not discussed, but HIV/AIDS disrupts the privacy of intimate relations and sheds unwelcome light on social taboos. Many of those who are HIV-positive already belong to socially vulnerable groups, such as men who have sex with men, commercial sex workers, or intravenous drug users. Because of the social implications, including fear of stigmatization and ostracism, many Africans choose not to be tested to learn their HIV status (a phenomenon that is not unique to Africa, of course). In recent years, progress has been made in decreasing the stigma associated with HIV/AIDS and other life-threatening diseases, as you will learn from the experiences highlighted in this book.

An Introduction to Health Systems and Structures in Africa

Most countries in the world have healthcare systems that differ substantially from that of the United States. To be effective in your global health work, you must understand the health system structure in your destination country. The following is a broad overview of the typical healthcare system in most African countries.

In the latter half of the twentieth century, many resource-limited countries developed national healthcare systems modeled after the health system in Britain. Administered by the government, these systems were designed to provide comprehensive services to the entire population. Unfortunately, for many reasons—shortfalls in funding, wavering political commitment, and competing priorities—most governments have been unable to provide the desired comprehensive package of healthcare services for all their citizens. Consequently, several parallel service providers and entities have emerged to fill the gaps: private-sector health facilities, NGOs, and faith-based organizations (FBOS; see the glossary). There are also individuals, groups, and other entities involved in the provision of healthcare or public health services, most often at the community level, who form part of the informal health system; these informal caregivers include family members, traditional birth attendants working outside the formal health sector, unlicensed traditional healers, and pharmacists or drug dispensers (whose advice on medications is often sought).

The healthcare system in a typical African country—indeed, in most countries around the world—is organized under a national Ministry of Health (MOH). Departments within the ministry address key health issues such as the regulation and oversight of public hospitals, preventive care services, and maternal and child health. The ministry is responsible for both public health services and direct patient care services. Most health facilities—from large, tertiary care referral hospitals (usually situated in large urban areas) to the smallest health clinic or outpost—are part of the public-sector national healthcare system. Most healthcare providers are employed by the government, and work at public healthcare facilities where care is generally provided free of charge. However, patients may have to pay fees for diagnostic tests such as a chest x-rays, laboratory tests, and prescribed medications. In many countries, national policy dictates that children under age five and pregnant women are exempt from these fees and receive all care free of charge.

Because the public health facilities—charged with the provision of care to the entire populace—are often understaffed and underfunded, many patients seek care in the private sector. Private-sector services also can range from relatively large hospitals to private doctors' offices. Private laboratories and pharmacies also exist to fill the gaps left by insufficient public-sector facilities. In many settings, healthcare workers—particularly doctors—work in both the private and the public sectors. Often physicians will work during usual business hours at a public facility and spend evenings and weekends at a private clinic, perhaps in their home, attending to patients on a fee-for-service basis. This allows public-sector healthcare providers to supplement their public salaries, which are often low.

Healthcare is delivered in a variety of facilities, from large, centralized national hospitals to smaller, local level facilities. Typically, the most sophisticated level of healthcare is provided by the national referral hospital, which is often affiliated with the national medical school, if the country has one. The next level of care is available at regional or district hospitals that vary in size and capacity, and that may include outpatient clinics. There may be sub-district facilities, which most commonly are outpatient facilities. The most basic level of care is delivered at health clinics or health outposts, often located in rural areas and providing care to people living in remote locations. Such facilities in remote locations often face special challenges. Sometimes they lack the basic tools of medical diagnosis and care, which can compromise the scope and sometimes the quality of care. The difficulties of terrain and inefficient drug distribution networks can result in limited access to appropriate medications in rural areas. Lack of resources and low government salaries in such challenging settings sometimes lead to frustration and irregular work attendance on the part of the healthcare workers. Some rural health facilities or outposts have acquired a bad reputation, and rural residents are often wary or distrustful of the quality of care they will receive there. Consequently, many patients will bypass their nearest local healthcare facility and seek care directly at a district, regional, or even national-level facility. In some countries, deliberate attention is being paid to building a cadre of community health workers to deliver specific aspects of healthcare in the home and community, such as first-line management of malaria and common childhood illnesses. The description of community-based care in the Rwanda chapter is a good example.

Many of the country chapters that follow will discuss the impact of three leading infectious diseases in Africa—HIV/AIDS, TB, and malaria. In many African countries, efforts to address these health threats are organized under the country's ministry of health through what are termed vertical disease programs (that is, programs aimed at diagnosing and treating a specific disease). These programs, usually named the National AIDS Control Program, the National TB (and often Leprosy) Control Program, and the National Malaria Control Program, are organized to respond to the respective disease by addressing both public health aspects of disease control in the community and patient care aspects, including the diagnosis and treatment of individuals with the disease. As a result, patients with possible TB can go to the TB clinic to have their sputum analyzed; if they are diagnosed with TB, they will be assigned to a TB clinic where they will be monitored and receive their TB medicines—but only their TB medicines—free of charge, due to the public health threat of untreated TB. Similarly, a patient could go to a testing center for HIV and, if found to be HIV-infected, would receive care and treatment with antiretrovirals in an HIV care and treatment center. Although other common HIV-associated opportunistic infections may be diagnosed and treated at specialized HIV clinics, the clinics do not provide all primary care services. Having specialized care clinics has both advantages (for instance, the quality of care is often higher, since care is focused on a specific disease) and disadvantages (for instance, care becomes fragmented, since patients must visit separate clinics to cover all their healthcare needs). The common occurrence of dual infection with HIV and TB has galvanized efforts to integrate care between these two historically different disease control programs. Attempts at integrated care for these conditions are described in the South Africa chapter.

Most country chapters in this book provide an overview of the country's healthcare system and infrastructure and discuss major initiatives that address the country's critical health issues.

Significant Health Issues in Africa

Many chapters of this book appear to emphasize HIV/AIDS, TB, and malaria as the leading health issues in the African countries discussed. This is because of the huge burdens that these diseases represent on the population, their disruption to national economies and family structures, and the undoubted international attention that the increasing incidence of these diseases has roused. In addition, many of the authors who contributed to this book have special expertise and many years of experience in infectious disease management and treatment. However, many chapters also call your attention to a range of other pressing issues in Africa: child health needs (in the Rwanda and Tanzania chapters); traffic accidents (in the Ghana chapter); malnutrition (in the Rwanda and Tanzania chapters); zoonoses (in the Uganda chapter); women's health and reproductive outcomes (in the Maghreb chapter); violence (in the South Africa and Maghreb chapters); and the insidious rise of chronic diseases among Africans (in the South Africa chapter). Limited funding for healthcare, infrastructure weaknesses that limit the provision of essential and basic health services, and severe shortages of the skilled human resources needed for adequate provision of healthcare are universal problems in African countries. Environmental degradation, limited resources for adequate personal and community sanitation, the inadequate availability of clean water and reliable energy resources, and limited transportation infrastructure and resources all impact health status and opportunities for improved health and well-being for many Africans. Although this book does not cover these issues in depth, the data provided at the conclusion of each country chapter will provide you insights into these issues and allow you to make comparisons among countries.

Global Health Efforts on an International Scale

International Organizations at Work in Africa

Throughout this book, you will find examples of the work of many agencies that carry out humanitarian, human rights, and global health activities in African countries. Many agencies choose a specific set of needs on which to focus their efforts, such as hunger, healthcare, education, human rights, protection and resettlement of refugees, clean water, and response to disasters and emergencies. The agencies include arms of the UN, like the World Health Organization (WHO; see the glossary); U.S. government agencies such as the United States Agency for International Development (USAID; see the glossary) and the President's Emergency Plan for AIDS Relief (PEPFAR; see the glossary); NGOS; and projects initiated by universities in the United States and other countries in collaboration with their African counterparts. Often these agencies and organizations act in collaboration. In each country chapter, the authors provide insights into organizations working in the country, and partnerships that carry out global health initiatives. Many key organizations at work in Africa are also described in the book's glossary.

Perhaps the most widely recognized initiative driving research and a focus on humanitarian issues today is the Gates Grand Challenges in Global Health. Bill Gates has said: "There is no bigger test for humanity than the crisis of global health."[16]

The Bill & Melinda Gates Foundation, in partnership with the U.S. National Institutes of Health, created the Grand Challenges initiative in 2003 to "identify critical scientific challenges in global health and increase research on diseases that cause millions of deaths in the developing world."[17] At the creation of the initiative, Bill Gates noted a remarkable disparity: a mere 10 percent of medical research is devoted to diseases that cause 90 percent of the world's overall health burden. He concluded that "the world is failing billions."[18] The health problems that disproportionately affect the world's poorest people — malaria, TB, HIV/AIDS, and malnutrition — had been receiving relatively little attention in the world of medical research. Gates created the Grand Challenges in Global Health to intentionally direct funds and research interest, and engage minds from many disciplines on the most critical challenges in global health.

The Gates idea of grand challenges is modeled on the concept of critical unsolved problems put forth by the German mathematician David Hilbert in 1900. In mathematics, Hilbert's articulation of unsolved problems is credited with driving innovation and problem solving even into the present. Similarly, the Gates Foundation has challenged researchers to address unsolved problems that stand in the way of progress toward improving global health. The challenges include seven long-term goals to improve health in developing countries. They are to:

Improve childhood vaccines;
Create new vaccines;
Control insects that transmit agents of disease;
Improve nutrition to promote health;
Improve drug treatment of infectious diseases to limit drug
   resistance;
Cure latent and chronic infections; and
Measure disease and health status accurately and economically
   in developing countries.

The first round of Grand Challenge funding ($200 million in 2005) supported forty-three diverse projects, and the most recent round of funding (May 2009) is supporting eighty-one projects (at $100,000 each) that address innovative ways to improve health in developing countries. The Gates' humanitarian initiative distinguishes challenges from problems. At the core of the distinction is the recognition that progress in addressing the problems of human suffering in the developing regions of the world will come not merely from scientific discovery, but also from the application of research results to reduce inequities. The challenges that have been articulated point directly at the results that need to be achieved. They remind us that global health encompasses prevention as well as treatment of disease and is deeply interwoven with politics, economics, policy, and human behavior.

A Framework for Global Improvement:
The UN Millennium Development Goals
A useful framework from which to envision and measure global improvement in social justice, education, economic well-being, and health is contained in the UN Millennium Development Goals (MDGs).[19] The Millennium Declaration, adopted by 189 nations at the UN Millennium Summit in 2000, set the actions and targets that became the eight MDGs. These goals set social development and health objectives to reduce extreme poverty and disease in the world. They do so by addressing the world's major challenges in economic development, social justice, and health, with achievement targets for the year 2015. The eight broad goals are:

Goal 1: Eradicate extreme poverty and hunger;
Goal 2: Achieve universal primary education;
Goal 3: Promote gender equality and empower women;
Goal 4: Reduce child mortality;
Goal 5: Improve maternal health;
Goal 6: Combat HIV/AIDS, malaria, and other diseases;
Goal 7: Ensure environmental sustainability; and
Goal 8: Develop a global partnership for development.

The MDGs recognize the interdependence among reducing poverty, ensuring social justice, empowering individuals, removing disparities, improving health, and working toward sustainable development. Inherent in the articulation of these goals for global improvement is the ability to track changes and progress over time. Progress toward the goals is being measured by tracking sixty pre-defined indicators. For instance, the first target for Goal 1 (eradicate extreme poverty and hunger) is to cut in half, between the baseline year 1990 and 2015, the proportion of people whose income is less than $1 a day. Thus, the proportion of people in a country or region living on less than $1 a day is the indicator for tracking progress toward this goal.

Progress Toward the Goals: Where Are We Now?
In a report published in 2007, the midway point between 2000 and 2015 in tracking the MDGs, the assessment for many African countries appears disheartening.[20] Major gains have been made in some countries in such areas as education and the prevention and management of HIV/AIDS. However, the analysis points to the conclusion that most African countries have not been able to make sufficient progress toward eradicating extreme poverty and its effects. In sub-Saharan Africa in particular, the current assessment is that none of the goals will be achieved.

For each of the countries in this book you can find current information, including selected MDG indicators, in the section titled "Country Data" at the conclusion of each country chapter. These data will give you a glimpse at the country's current status and allow country-to-country comparisons.

As we have seen, the scope of humanitarian action and global health can be very broad. To those contemplating humanitarian and global health undertakings, we think it's important to remember that good deeds come in all sizes. One individual's small contributions can indeed have a big impact.

NOTES

1. The quoted phrase appears in two United Nations documents, the 1948 Universal Declaration of Human Rights (http://www.un.org/en/documents/udhr/index.shtml) and the 1966 International Covenant on Civil and Political Rights (http://www2.ohchr.org/english/law/ccpr.htm).

2. Information about the Albert Schweitzer Fellowship program is available at http://www.schweitzerfellowship.org.

3. Øivind Stenersen, "The Humanitarian Nobel Peace Prizes," 26 February 2004. (http://nobelprize.org/nobel_prizes/peace/articles/stenersen/index.html).

4. Social legislation in the United States includes the laws that enacted

programs such as Social Security, Medicare, and Medicaid; provided workers' compensation and unemployment benefits; protected voters' rights; and banned child labor.

5. International Federation of Red Cross and Red Crescent Societies, "Principles and Values: Humanitarian Values" (http://www.ifrc.org/what/values/).

6. The Red Cross/NGO Code of Conduct. International Federation of Red Cross and Red Crescent Societies, 1994. (http://www.ifrc.org/publicat/conduct/code.asp) or (http://www.ifrc.org/publicat/conduct/).

7. The principle of neutrality was intentionally left out of the Red Cross/NGO Code because some nongovernmental humanitarian agencies are committed to working on issues of justice and human rights while simultaneously providing impartial humanitarian assistance.

8. Centers for Disease Control and Prevention, "2009 H1N1 Flu. Situation Update," 11 August 2010. (http://www.cdc.gov/h1n1flu/).

9. Roland Oliver, and J. D. Fage, *A Short History of Africa*, 6th ed. (New York: Penguin, 1990), 101.

10. Ibid., 102.

11. Abderrahmane Sissako, director, *Bamako*, New York: Louverture Films, (2006).

12. Paul Farmer, "On Suffering and Structural Violence: A View from Below," in *Issues on Social Suffering*, ed. A. Kleinman, V. Das, and M. Lock (a special issue of *Daedalus, Journal of American Academy of Arts and Sciences* 125, no. 1 (winter 1996): 261–83).

13. Paul Farmer, *Infections and Inequalities: The Modern Plagues* (Berkeley: University of California Press, 2001) p.79.

14. Rachel King, "Collaboration with Traditional Healers in HIV/AIDS Prevention and Care in Sub-Saharan Africa: A Literature Review" (Geneva: UNAIDS, September 2000; http://data.unaids.org/Publications/IRC-pub01/jc299-tradheal_en.pdf).

15. One example of a medical university that offers training in traditional healing is Muhimbili University of Health and Allied Sciences, in Tanzania.

16. Bill Gates, "Global Health Is Humanity's Challenge."(Speech at the World Health Organization, Fifty-eighth World Health Assembly. Geneva, Switzerland, 16 May 2005. http://www.paho.org/English/DD/PIN/ptoday07_sep05.htm).

17. Bill & Melinda Gates foundation website. (http://www.gatesfoundation.org/press-releases/Pages/grant-for-grand-challenges-in-global-health-030126.aspx).

18. Bill Gates, "Global Health Is Humanity's Challenge." (Speech at the World Health Organization, Fifty-eighth World Health Assembly, 16 May 2005) Op.cit.

19. United Nations, "The Millennium Development Goals Report 2005"

(New York: United Nations, 2005; http://unstats.un.org/unsd/mi/pdf/MDG
%20Book.pdf).

20. United Nations, "The Millennium Development Goals Report 2007"
(New York: United Nations, 2007; http://www.un.org/millenniumgoals/pdf/
mdg2007.pdf).

SUGGESTED READING OR VIEWING

Jong, Elaine C., and Christopher Sanford, editors. *The Travel and Tropical Medicine Manual.* 4th ed. Philadelphia: Saunders/Elsevier, 2008.

Kidder, Tracy. *Mountains beyond Mountains.* New York: Random House, 2003.

MDG [Millennium Development Goals] Monitor. http://www.mdgmonitor.org/
map.cfm?goal=0&indicator=0&cd= (The website allows you to track progress
toward the goals using the set indicators and offers excellent visual tools and
maps that highlight progress in Africa).

Oliver, Roland, and J. D. Fage. *A Short History of Africa.* 6th ed. New York:
Penguin, 1990.

O'Neil, Edward Jr. *A Practical Guide to Global Health Service.* Chicago: American
Medical Association, 2006.

O'Neil, Edward, Jr. *Awakening Hippocrates: A Primer on Health, Poverty and
Global Service* (paperback). Chicago: American Medical Association, 2006.

Sissako, Abderrahmane, director. *Bamako.* New York: Louverture Films, 2006

The MDG Africa Steering Group. Achieving the Millennium Development Goals
in Africa. http://www.mdgafrica.org/ and www.uneca.org/cfm/2008/docs/
AssessingProgressinAfricaMDGs.pdf.

United Nations. "Millennium Development Goals Reports," published annually.
New York: United Nations Department of Public Information. http://www.un
.org/millenniumgoals/.

LISA V. ADAMS

LAUREL A. SPIELBERG

STEPHANIE WILLMAN BORDAT

SAIDA KOUZZI

JOYCE A. SACKEY

NAMEETA M. DOOKERAN

STELLA SAFO

ELIZABETH A. TALBOT

TIPS FOR TRAVELERS TO AFRICA

In preparing for your African travels, you will want to maximize your ability to work successfully in the culture of your destination country and minimize potential sources of stress during your travels. This chapter offers some suggestions for accomplishing both goals. Undoubtedly, you will find yourself in an environment unlike any you have been in before, unless you already have many years of experience in low-income, resource-poor countries. For many travelers to Africa, the most pressing questions are: "Will I be able to accomplish what I set out to do?" and "What will it be like?"

With the aim of helping you understand the African context and achieve what you set out to do, we first offer some suggestions for working in African countries. Many of these suggestions have to do with realistically aligning your expectations to the culture you will experience. Whatever your destination, you will want to establish positive relationships with the diverse stakeholders at work there, and work appropriately and effectively with your colleagues and other people with whom you come in contact.

Working Successfully and Effectively in an African Culture

You will quickly become aware of the huge disparities in resources and standards of living between your home country and most African countries.[1] You should also realize that there are huge disparities in resource distribution and standards of living within countries,[2] particularly between urban and rural areas in most of Africa. Urban areas often develop economically and socially at a faster pace and benefit from development initiatives that have not reached more remote areas. For example, a newly developed drug or medical treatment may be heavily promoted and highlighted in a country. You may find that it is widely distributed and available in cities, but remains unavailable in the countryside where clinics and outposts may have only the most basic medicines in stock. Similarly, government health education and awareness messages, such as those encouraging women to give birth in hospitals, may be unrealistic for rural residents. Women living in remote and rural areas may not have time, transportation, or money to travel several hours to the nearest town with a hospital in order to give birth.

While recognizing that regional and urban-rural disparities exist, you should not necessarily presume that people will differ in their behavior and beliefs based on geographic residence or standard of living. Don't assume, for instance, that people in rural or disadvantaged areas have more conservative views on social issues or stricter standards for behavior than people in urban or more privileged areas.

Gender and ethnicity impact health and access to healthcare in every culture. It will be important for you to try to determine what impact gender and ethnicity have on health and healthcare in your destination country. In most countries, women are more likely to be illiterate than men. In many countries, and particularly in rural areas, women may speak only the local dialect, while men may also speak English, French, Arabic, or whatever is the official language of business, trade, and education. Women may not be comfortable with the typically all-male staff at public health centers and clinics, and therefore may avoid seeking prenatal or other care specific to their own health needs. Women often seek care only for their children, such as immunizations, or for other concerns that their husbands — who typically control the household resources — deem important. In many cultures, although married women may be able to obtain birth control pills at public health clinics, doctors may not explain their use sufficiently, and women may not be able to read the written instructions. Power dynamics within households may limit the effectiveness of awareness-raising activities targeted to women. For example, outreach to women on sexual and reproductive matters is often ineffective if there is no corresponding outreach and education to the men.

People often deny that certain problems or sensitive issues exist in their communities. For example, they may deny that HIV/AIDS is a problem in their own town or village. It is not uncommon in communities in the Maghreb, for instance, for people to say that HIV/AIDS only affects people who have sex outside of marriage, and since everyone in their community is a "good Muslim," they aren't affected or at risk. Sometimes, too, doctors at local health clinics may compromise science and healthcare to help patients save face, particularly in small communities. For instance, anecdotal reports describe doctors telling women with sexually transmitted diseases (STDS) that they just need to wash themselves more, since telling a wife she has an STD would imply that her husband is an adulterer, causing both of them shame. The illegality of certain topics in some settings and the potential for ostracism make it difficult for people to discuss some topics. Thus, it may be more difficult than you hope to collect seemingly valid data for research, if what you are seeking are hard, quantitative facts. However, as you explore, inquire, and absorb what you see and hear, remember that the anecdotal and qualitative information you may be able to collect can be more rich and valid (as well as easier to obtain) than quantitative data.

At other times, you will be surprised at what people are willing to share with you. Try to avoid preconceptions about what is taboo and what is not in your destination culture. People may talk indirectly and guardedly about sensitive topics if they don't know you, or if they think you are talking to them in some kind of official capacity. You will need to think about the best way to navigate taboo issues carefully and sensitively. In most places, you are likely to find that people can be extremely open and direct when talking about most issues—even very sensitive ones—to others of their own age and gender. For example, if you are a young woman, you may feel excluded from an old boys' network among government officials, but you may be able to have quite frank and open discussions with other young woman. It is not so much what you talk about that is taboo and sensitive, but how you go about it that makes it taboo or not, and that can make or break your credibility. In other words, it is not the topics that can offend so much as the way of talking about them and with whom you discuss them.

If your work involves gaining access to information or statistics, you might find that the information you seek will not be easily available or readily provided to you. The credible, solid information that you want simply may not exist, or you may require a number of administrative authorizations to obtain it, or people may not feel comfortable sharing it for a host of reasons. International visitors frequently arrive in a country and ask for statistics that simply do not exist. Sometimes it may be easier and quicker to gain the information you need by working at the local level or with nongovernmental organizations (NGOS; see the glossary) rather than approaching central government bureaucracies in the capital city. You should always be aware that social, political, and religious considerations may influence supposedly scientific endeavors and the way information is presented. For example, surveys in some cultures may avoid direct questions on sensitive issues like abortion. Official government campaigns may present information with socially acceptable but inaccurate language. Expectations about proper behavior may affect people's assumptions and therefore their behavior, resulting in distorted or otherwise inaccurate information. For example, medical personnel in some settings may not consider pregnancy as a possibility when an unmarried woman comes to a clinic with certain symptoms. Again, we remind you of the value of qualitative information.

You should be conscious of the fact that in many societies where there is a sense of social stratification—whether based on gender, ethnicity, education, or income—your ability to work effectively with people may depend on your age and marital status. Your age and how much experience you are perceived to have will affect how people view the legitimacy of your knowledge, how much knowledge you can impart, and how much work you can get done. Be prepared to have the most credibility and be the most effective with people of your own age and marital status.

You and the organization, agency, educational or religious institution that you represent are certainly not alone in working in Africa. You should be aware that many Africans may have had experiences with international development organizations that give money or build infrastructure; people may be less familiar with development work focused on capacity-building, grassroots-education, and raising awareness of health and other issues. It may take extra work on your part to help people understand how you differ from representatives of other organizations they've experienced in the past.

People initially may be wary of you and your work; they may not consider researchers or volunteer workers as neutral, objective, impartial, and well-meaning. People may make assumptions about you, your agenda, and your morality based on the issue you are working on, and they may or may not help you with your work depending on whether or not they agree or identify with you. Make a special effort to explain your work clearly and seek input from your co-workers in the country to ensure that you are not inadvertently presenting yourself in a way that could be misinterpreted. The friendships you develop with people within the country will allow you opportunities for frank discussions about how you can be effective in your role, given your status as an outsider.

Working in another culture can be frustrating at times. Things may not happen on the same schedule and at the same pace that you are used to at home. Be prepared to feel frustrated; you may not see the results of your work immediately, or even during the time you are in Africa. Change is a slow process, and you may not be present to see the fruits of your efforts. As your planning and work proceed, you may need to revise your work plan, project expectations, and time frames for getting things accomplished. Inevitably, things will take longer than you originally anticipate or may be used to. It is best not to enter your project with too rigid a schedule or strategy. If your work requires ministerial or other official government authorizations, or your research needs institutional review board (IRB) approval, be advised that this process could take months. If your personal work style is very product-oriented and outcome-driven, you may have to reduce your expectations and become more sensitive to process and procedural matters. Remember that accomplishing your objectives is a long-term process that will require commitment, trust, and sustainable relationships. Flexibility and patience are likely to be the two most important traits you will need to cultivate during your overseas work.

You will also need to become informed of and sensitive to the most appropriate and effective way to contact people for meetings or to gain information in your destination country. Meeting with people in person is always a necessary first step. Don't expect to be able to do much pre-liminary communication or work by e-mail or telephone before arriving in the country. Indeed, be prepared for a lot of unanswered phone calls and e-mail messages. You will have to be politely persistent until you get face-to-face meetings for introductions, which you will need before you can start building the basis for future relationships.

Personal relationships and contacts are essential in setting up meet-ings and getting to know the people who will be most critical to your work. If you want to meet someone, it's best to find a person you've come to know who can personally introduce you, rather than sending a cold e-mail or fax or just showing up. Personal relationships are very important; you are most likely to be granted access to information and be able to accomplish your work if you use a contact-based approach.

Generally speaking, dress codes for work are more formal in African cultures than in the United States. You should bring somewhat more formal clothing than you may be used to for work settings: button-down shirts or polo shirts for men, and long skirts or loose-fitting pants or capris for women are suitable. Never wear shorts in a professional setting. For official meetings and other professional gatherings men should be prepared to wear a shirt and tie, and women a skirt or dress, even in very hot and humid conditions. Because of the heat, synthetic materials are preferable as they dry faster and are generally cooler. To help guide you in how much to pack, you should ask whether you will have access to laundry facilities or the ability to wash your own clothes at your destination site. In addition to dressing more formally, consider dressing conservatively, especially in more religiously conservative set-tings. We advise women to avoid sleeveless tops and skirts or dresses that end above the knee. Shorts and tank tops can be worn if you plan to travel on your own, but not to work or to a meeting. The more conser-vatively you dress, the less attention you will draw to yourself as an out-sider. A suggested packing list is included at the end of this chapter.

Finally, be sensitive to the fact that bribery, corruption, and gift giv-ing can affect many areas of life in Africa, including the health sector. As an example, a study carried out by Transparency Maroc[3] concluded that in Morocco, the health sector was perceived as the third most plagued by corruption; 40 percent of people surveyed who had had contact with health sector personnel in the previous year had paid a bribe to them. In 59 percent of those cases, the bribe was paid for access to a public service—to obtain a right legally guaranteed by the law—such as an appointment for a medical examination, admission to a hospital, or to obtain treatment.

Some Practical Considerations for Working in a Clinical Setting

Before arriving in your African destination, particularly if you are going to work on a health-related project, you may find it helpful to review material such as the country's essential medicines list, standard treatment guidelines, and other information published by the country's ministry of health or other government health agencies, all of which is usually available online.[4] If you will be involved in direct patient care, it is best to bring your own basic medical equipment—including a blood pressure cuff, stethoscope, otoscope, and ophthalmoscope—since some of these items may be in short supply among local healthcare providers. Keep a flashlight handy in case of electrical power outages and for when you are traveling or working late. If you will be seeing patients in rural settings, consider carrying an ample supply of antibacterial, alcohol-based hand sanitizer.[5]

Essential Planning Tips for Your African Travels

Planning your trip will require advance preparation, both in terms of practical tasks and educating yourself on your destination and the project you propose to carry out. The following tips focus on activities that we consider essential before you go. So don't leave home without. . . .

Familiarizing Yourself with Your Destination Country

Once you have committed yourself to a destination and a project in Africa, we encourage you to use your time wisely before you depart: learn about the people, place, and culture of your destination, and memorize at least basic greetings in the local language or languages. These efforts will prove well worth the time once you arrive in the country. Reading the chapter on your country in this book is a good place to start. Supplement your research with the suggested readings or films listed. Taking courses in medical anthropology, African history, politics, and culture (ideally, those tailored to the country or region to which you are traveling) can expand your understanding of the social, historical, and political context in which you will be working. This knowledge and background can make you more effective in your global health work.

Many established sites and programs that host volunteers and students will provide specific travel guides or orientation documents—be sure to ask about them. Recently updated travel books and the Internet can be good resources for practical details such as accommodations, restaurants, markets, and Internet cafes. However, nothing takes the place of speaking to someone who has been to the country, city, town, or village where you will be working. Talking to nationals from your destination country can be very helpful; you should seek out international students from that country, and see if there is an immigrant community or organization you can contact. If there are students at your school from the country you are going to, or previous volunteers from your host organization you can contact, ask them about their experience, and any advice they can offer or lessons learned, and get as many nitty-gritty details as you can about what your daily life will be like in Africa. Such contacts can also help you refine the recommended packing list at the end of this chapter, separating essential from non-essential items for your trip. Travel books and orientation guides may also provide packing lists.[6]

The U.S. State Department provides vital information for anyone traveling to Africa. Its website gives country-specific details of travel requirements, safety tips, and warnings.[7]

Getting Your Passport and Necessary Visas
Many countries require you to obtain your visa in advance. Even if the country will issue you a visa when you arrive, it is convenient to have this taken care of before you depart. Be sure to allow enough time if you do get your visa in the United States. It typically takes at least two weeks to process your visa application, so it is best to start this process a month before you depart. If you expect to travel in and out of your destination country during your stay, inquire whether you can obtain a multi-entry visa or can get additional visas issued at the borders you will cross. Contacting the embassy of your destination country (in Washington, D.C. if you reside in the U.S. or in Ottawa if you reside in Canada) will provide you with the most up-to-date information on passport, visa, and other requirements. Some African countries have

consulates in other large U.S. or Canadian cities, such as New York, Chicago, Los Angeles, Toronto, or Vancouver, and many also allow you to apply for a visa online. The embassy's website should have information about visas under its consular services section, and many have a visa application you can download. Some countries require you to have a work visa if you are going to work while there. Information on work visas is available from the country's embassy or ministry of immigration website. If you intend to travel from one country to another in Africa, be sure to inquire at each embassy about any special requirements that will affect you as you enter or leave a country. A passport that will not expire for at least six months is usually required for entry into any African country. Be sure to check the expiration date of your passport and renew it before you travel if it is due to expire within six months. As with visas, it can take several weeks to renew a passport.

Be sure to make copies of your passport identification page (the page with your photo) and any other important documents such as your health insurance, evacuation insurance (see below), and contacts and numbers of how you can be reached in the country(ies) where you will be staying. Keep these copies separate from the originals. Also, leave a copy with a relative or friend back home.

Visiting a Travel Clinic

Travel clinics are an essential source of health guidance before you travel, and you should be sure to seek medical advice before traveling to any African destination. In fact, we consider this a mandatory step for all our students traveling overseas. Travel clinics are staffed by health professionals with expertise in infectious disease and travel medicine. In preparation for your trip, a travel clinic can provide you with pre-travel counseling, advice on food and water precautions while you travel, immunizations you will need for the countries you are visiting, and prescriptions for malaria prophylaxis if indicated, and can recommend medicines and supplies you should carry with you. Be sure to obtain a yellow fever immunization card if you are traveling to an area where yellow fever is endemic,[8] or to obtain a medical waiver if immunization is not indicated or is medically contraindicated in your case. This documentation is issued only by a yellow fever center, such as some travel clinics. Carry this documentation with you within your passport; this is especially important and often required for entry into a neighboring country where yellow fever is not endemic if you are traveling from a yellow fever area. There is no yellow fever transmission in the most northern and southern countries of Africa, but yellow fever does occur in the central Africa region.

It is particularly important to understand the risk of malaria in your destination country or countries and to begin malaria prophylaxis before you enter an area where malaria is endemic. Effective antimalarial drugs may not be available once you arrive at your destination; you should bring with you an adequate supply for your entire trip. Insect precautions—including insect repellents for exposed skin, long-sleeved clothing, insecticide-treated clothes and bed nets—are critical to avoid malaria, as well as other vector-borne diseases such as dengue and tick-borne rickettsial diseases. The Centers for Disease Control and Prevention (CDC) recommends using an insect repellent that contains DEET (a 30 percent concentration is typical), Picaridin, oil of lemon eucalyptus, or IR3535 on exposed skin.[9] Long sleeves and socks should be worn in the evenings. Long pants with shirt tucked in and closed-toe shoes are advised for hiking. Travelers to malaria endemic areas should always sleep under an insecticide-treated bed net. Find out before you depart whether your destination housing has bed nets or you should bring your own. Many sporting-goods stores sell both bed nets and clothing treated with an insecticide (usually permethrin).

In addition, you should be aware of the risk of schistosomiasis (often called bilharzia in Africa; see the glossary), a fascinating and avoidable disease transmitted by a parasite that penetrates your skin during even brief contact with fresh water. Even though locals will often encourage you to swim, assuring you that bilharzia is not present, it is wise to avoid swimming in non-chlorinated fresh water (that is, any lake or river) throughout Africa.[10]

Travel clinics also provide post-travel counseling, and diagnosis and treatment of illnesses acquired abroad. Some diseases, such as malaria, may not become apparent until after you return from your trip. If you experience symptoms that are prolonged or unusual, or were exposed to fresh water in an area where schistosomiasis is endemic, get a post-travel checkup at a travel or tropical medicine clinic.

The CDC provides useful information about international travel on its website. You can click your destination on a world map and learn about travel and immunization recommendations, health precautions, recommended medications and supplies to take with you, and how to seek healthcare in your destination country. Although never a substitute for a full pre-travel evaluation in a travel clinic, the CDC website can help you locate travel clinics in every state.[11] Student health services at many colleges and universities provide travel advice, immunizations, and medical information for students traveling abroad, and many medical centers have travel clinics. Be sure to contact your student health service or travel clinic at least one month before your departure date, as some immunizations require multiple doses given at intervals, and it is best to receive as many doses as possible before you depart. In addition, you will need time to fill prescriptions and purchase some items that may be recommended, such as an insecticide-treated bed net or clothing. However, even if your departure date is imminent, a travel clinic can still provide you with essential advice and at least some of the services you will need on short notice.

Getting Recommended Medications before You Go

At right is a list of medications that a clinic or other provider may prescribe or recommend that you take with you. Be sure to carry all medicines in your carry-on luggage during your travels and keep them in a secure place in your accommodations.

Making Sure You Have Insurance Coverage: Health and Evacuation

Be sure to check your health insurance policy to learn what coverage you have during travel abroad. If you do not have health insurance, you should make arrangements for coverage for the months you will be away. We also recommend purchasing medical evacuation coverage through a well-established company such as International SOS.[12] Many schools and universities will provide medical evacuation coverage for their students when they are overseas, so if you are a student, check first with the appropriate international or health office at your school.

Evacuation insurance is not the same as health insurance: evacuation insurance will handle all the logistics in case you need to be evacuated out of a country for medical reasons. However, it does not cover the provision of care at the facility to which you are evacuated. Therefore, you will need both health insurance and evacuation coverage. The U.S. Department of State website provides an assessment of the adequacy of medical facilities within foreign countries, and it often gives advice as to whether medical treatment can be sought within a country or evacuation is advised.[13] Evacuation coverage for all travelers is a high priority, since ability to pay is usually a determinant of whether you will receive medical transportation services.

Making Sure You will Have Enough Money

Before you depart, it is important to ensure that you will have adequate access to money while you are overseas. You should try to find out if you will be able to obtain and exchange cash or traveler's checks in the country or countries you will be visiting. Many large urban areas have ATMS from which you can access a U.S. bank account, although they often charge a fee. Traveler's checks provide the security that if stolen or lost they can be replaced, but in our experience they can be exchanged only at limited sites (usually just large hotels and some banks) and always at a much lower exchange rate than U.S. currency. Money can be wired through Western Union offices for a fee; investigating this option before you go may be useful in case you have an unexpected or emergency need for additional cash.

Major hotels usually accept credit cards. In some settings, exchange offices and banks refuse to exchange older or crumpled bills, so it is best to travel with newer, crisp bills whenever possible. Many travelers find they get the best exchange rates if they use US $100 bills issued no later than 2000. Some exchange agencies will give a lower rate for bills in denominations under $50, regardless of the total amount you exchange. Again, your host organization or previous volunteers can provide advice on these issues.

Health and Environmental Hazards

Waterborne illnesses are a common threat to travelers in settings where sanitation is compromised and access to clean water is limited. There are many forms of water purification or sterilization, including filters, heat, and chemical disinfection. Bottled water has become the main source of reliable water for travelers in Africa and can now be found in all urban and even some rural areas. While bottled water is undoubtedly most convenient for travelers, reliance on bottled water is creating a significant ecological problem, since most resource-limited countries do not recycle plastic bottles. You should plan carefully to find a reliable means of obtaining clean water throughout your stay. Travelers, especially those going to rural areas, may want to pack iodine or chlorine tablets for circumstances when they need to treat their own water. Further information on clean water and waterborne illnesses is available on the traveler's health pages of the CDC's website.[14]

Similarly, you should take precautions with food. Avoid uncooked fruits and vegetables, but if you must eat raw fruit, fruits that can be peeled are considered safer. In general, food that is thoroughly cooked under sanitary conditions is safest. We recommend that you do not purchase food from street vendors. It is best to get advice from other international volunteers or co-workers on recommended and trusted restaurants or carry-out (often called take-away) places. Travel books and Internet sites also list reliable restaurants for popular destinations.

During your time in Africa, you may find yourself invited to co-workers' or friends' homes for meals. These social invitations can raise uncertainty if you don't know how the food was prepared. To avoid seeming rude or unappreciative you will have to use your best judgment in deciding whether to accept small amounts of food. It's best to restrict your choices to thoroughly cooked items, while showing your sincere appreciation for the generous invitation and food offered.

Safety and Security

Up-to-date information about security concerns for travelers to any African country can be obtained from the U.S. State Department.[15] At the time of this writing, civil unrest is unusual in the countries profiled in this book. The crime rate in most cities in Africa is similar to that in any large urban area. Petty street crime and crimes of opportunity do occur. Pickpocketing, home invasions, "smash and grabs" from vehicles, and cell phone thefts, sometimes at knifepoint, are routinely reported to the police in many cities. Visitors should use care when talking on a cell phone — something it is best not to do while walking through urban areas. Urban areas can be particularly dangerous at night, and you may be advised to avoid walking in particular neighborhoods after dark. Common sense and usual street smarts are always advised. For example, women should not travel alone at night. Pay careful attention to and heed U.S. State Department warnings about unrest that may pose a special risk to travelers in particular areas or roads.

Sometimes items are stolen from baggage in transit between regions of a country or when traveling country-to-country within Africa. Never place any valuables (such as computers, cell phones, or expensive jewelry) in checked luggage at airports. In addition, roughly one in ten of our student travelers to Tanzania, for instance, experiences lost or delayed luggage. Be sure to have at least a change of clothes as well as all essential medicines, contact numbers, and critical electronic items with you in your carry-on bags.

Traffic and Transport

Driving in many African countries is challenging and risky.[16] In many countries that were British colonies or protectorates during their colonial period, traffic circulates on the left. The vast majority of roads in Africa, even in major cities, are unpaved. In some areas, roads are vulnerable to damage by heavy downpours in the rainy season. When traveling in rural areas, high speed limits, poor lighting, and roving game and domestic animals can make driving at night particularly hazardous. In many urban areas, public buses may be overloaded vehicles in poor condition, with untrained drivers, maneuvering crowded roads in poor conditions. You should try to determine the availability and safety of mini-van, taxi, and bus services in your destination country. Oftentimes, *moto-taxis*, *tro-tros*, and other informal means of transportation (which may be called different things in different countries) are inexpensive, but also hazardous. Motor vehicle accidents are a major cause of death and injury throughout Africa, so you should plan your ground transportation carefully.

When traveling by taxi, always negotiate the fare to your destination before you get in the car. If you are unsure about reasonable costs, it is best to ask co-workers or friends what the expected, reasonable fare is for your proposed trip. However, as a foreigner, you will probably be expected to pay a somewhat higher fare than a local resident.

Communication

Staying in touch with friends and family back home has been made much easier with the growing presence of Internet cafes and cell phone systems.

Cell Phones

Cell phones are widely used in most African countries. In fact, many African countries have leapfrogged telecommunications technology so the availability, line quality, and accessibility of cell phones are greater than that of landline phones. In each of the countries discussed in the book, the cell phone is the primary method of communication. Throughout many countries in Africa people are more likely to have cell phones than landlines. Many Africans rely heavily on text messaging rather than on the more time-consuming (and thus more costly) real-time conversations on their mobile phones.

You should ask about the best way to acquire a cell phone while in country. For instance, in Tanzania reasonably priced cell phones can be purchased at the airport, and a scratch-card system lets you add money to your account as needed. These scratch cards can be purchased at shops and kiosks on nearly every street corner in the larger cities. Consider borrowing or buying a basic cell phone if your own phone is not compatible with the use of locally available subscriber identity modules (SIM cards). Options for international calling include going to a tele-communication center (several are available in many towns), or making an online phone call from an Internet cafe or your own computer through software programs such as Skype.

Computers

If you plan to take a laptop or other electronic devices with you, you should buy appropriate plug adapters required for the different electrical sockets in your destination country. Be forewarned — not all electronic devices will be compatible with the 220-240 volts range used in African countries (as compared to the 110-120 volts range used in United States and Canada). For devices that are not compatible, you will need to buy a converter, which usually can also serve as a plug adapter. Be careful where you store electronic devices in hotel facilities or other areas — they are a temptation to thieves.

We strongly suggest that you back up your data regularly on a storage medium (such as a USB flash drive or external hard drive) that is kept in a separate location from your laptop in the event of laptop malfunction or theft. Although electricity is available in many towns and cities, there may be regular or occasional power outages. Thus, it is advisable to save your work often while using a laptop connected to an electrical power supply, and to consider using a surge protector.

Internet Access and E-mail

While Internet access is available in African countries, often through Internet cafes that cater to both locals and foreigners, Internet connection speeds may be somewhat slow, especially in less urban areas. In more remote areas, you may find Internet access only in select hotels.

An individual African's use of e-mail as a means of communication very much depends on his or her comfort with the technology, as well as on the availability, cost, and speed of Internet access. Thus, it is wise to ask your African collaborators about the best way to communicate with them in making preparations before your trip, as well as when you are in the country. Where Internet access is readily available, many travelers decide to maintain a blog to keep their friends and family updated on their activities. Keep in mind that postings on openly accessible tools (like blogs and YouTube) are public information; we strongly advise you to use group e-mails for information of a more personal nature and for comments that could be viewed as derogatory or critical of the location or the host organization.

We conclude this chapter with a recommended packing list of clothing and other essentials for your travels.

⊚ RECOMMENDED PACKING LIST

CLOTHING

T-shirts for men; blouses for women (the lighter weight, the better)
Collared or button-down shirts for men; blouses or tops that cover the shoulder for women (for work)
Jeans
Khakis for men; slacks, capris, or skirts for women (for work; lightweight is best)
Socks
Underwear
Comfortable walking shoes or sandals
An outfit or two for special events
Athletic shoes (optional)
Shower sandals (for example, flip-flops)
Pajamas
Bathing suit
Belt

Cold Weather Clothing and Hiking or Climbing Equipment

If you're going to southern Africa in the continent's winter or planning to do any climbing at high altitudes, you'll need the following items:

Winter jacket
Winter hat
Gloves

Long underwear

Hiking shoes (basic hiking gear can be rented in Africa)

OTHER ESSENTIALS

Passport (leave one photocopy with a trusted person at home and
bring several photocopies with you, keeping them in a separate
location from your passport)

Yellow immunization card or medical exemption (kept with your
passport)

Health insurance card

International evacuation insurance card

ATM card (to obtain cash in your destination country)

Cash for visa fee upon arrival (if required)

Insect repellent

Bedding (sheets or a sleeping bag)

Towel

Insecticide-treated bed net (if not available at your planned
accommodation)

Plug adapters

Cell phone

Camera

Personal toiletries

Hand sanitizer

Laptop

Binoculars

Flashlight (one that clips onto a key chain is handy)

Alarm clock

iPod (or other musical device)

Plastic bags for storing liquids and wet clothing

Multi-language dictionary (English and the language of your
destination country)

Travel journal

Extra duffel bag (for short trips and bringing purchases back home)

Small first-aid kit (with medications and bandages for minor injuries
like blisters)

Gifts for hosts (or anyone else you may visit)

1. The tips and advice in this section were contributed by Stephanie Willman Bordat and Saida Kouzzi, the authors of the Maghreb chapter. Their information for that region on this subject was so significant and relevant to working throughout Africa that the editors of this book asked them to expand the material for inclusion here.

2. It is important to acknowledge that great disparities in wealth, health, and access to healthcare also exist within the United States. Moreover, many of the useful tips in this chapter — such as avoiding making assumptions and how to approach sensitive topics — could be applied to working with different cultures, regional, and socioeconomic groups, within the United States. Cross-cultural issues arise at home as well as abroad, and you may find these tips equally helpful when you return to the United States.

3. Transparency Maroc, La corruption au Maroc: Synthèse des résultants des enquêtes d'intégrité. Casablanca, Morocco (2002). (http://www.transparency .org/contact_us/organisations/transparency_maroc). Transparency Maroc is the Moroccan arm of a global organization that works against corruption.

4. See, for example, World Health Organization, "Medicines Policy Documents from Selected African Countries" (http://collections.infocollections.org/ whocountry/en/cl/CL3.1.4/). This website includes essential medicines lists and standard treatment guidelines.

5. The information in this section on practical considerations was contributed by Joyce A. Sackey, Nameeta M. Dookeran, and Stella Safo, the authors of the Ghana chapter.

6. One good source of an extensive packing list is Garth Osborn and Patricia Ohmans, *Finding Work in Global Health: A Practical Guide for Jobseekers*, St. Paul, Minn.: Health Advocates, (2005).

7. See the U.S. Department of State home page, at http://www.state.gov/travel/.

8. You can determine where yellow fever is endemic by consulting the Centers for Disease Control and Prevention (CDC) website (http://wwwnc.cdc.gov/ travel/yellowbook/2010/chapter-2/yellow-fever.aspx).

9. Emily Zielinski-Gutierrez, Robert A. Wirtz, and Roger S. Nasci, "Protection against Mosquitoes, Ticks, and Other Insects and Arthropods," in CDC Health Information for International Travel ["The Yellow Book"] Atlanta, Ga.: Centers for Disease Control and Prevention, 2010; (http://wwwnc.cdc.gov/travel/ yellowbook/2010/chapter-2/protection-against-mosquitoes-ticks-insects -arthropods.aspx).

10. This important information on schistosomiasis and swimming precautions was contributed by Elizabeth A. Talbot, one of the authors of the Botswana chapter.

11. See http://www.cdc.gov/travel/.

12. See http://www.internationalsos.com.

13. See http://travel.state.gov/. By searching for your country destination on this website you can obtain useful advice on travel, safety, and healthcare in the country.

14. See http://wwwnc.cdc.gov/travel/.

15. See http://travel.state.gov/travel/cis_pa_tw/tw/tw_1764.html.

16. The material in this section was contributed by Joyce A. Sackey, Nameeta M. Dookeran, and Stella Safo, authors of the Ghana chapter.

ELIZABETH A. TALBOT

CHARLES WELLS

BARUDI MOSIMANEOTSILE

REPUBLIC OF BOTSWANA

Botswana is an enchanting place with wonderful people who are rising to meet great health challenges.

The Lay of the Land

Botswana is a stable, prosperous, democratic country in southern Africa that shares borders with Namibia, South Africa, Zambia and Zimbabwe. An area of 224,607 square miles (581,730 square kilometers), Botswana is the world's forty-seventh largest country, slightly smaller than Texas.[1] The Kalahari Desert comprises 70 percent of the country, and the climate throughout the country varies from arid to semi arid. High temperatures in January can routinely exceed 95°F (35°C), but it is the lows in June that seem to surprise visitors—on average 35°F (2°C). The Okavango Delta, the world's largest inland delta, is in the northwest of the country and is a major international tourist attraction. Other tourist attractions at which to view Botswana's diverse wildlife habitats include the Makgadikgadi Pan, a large salt pan in the north, and Chobe Game Park.

Botswana is divided into nine government districts, and the largest city is the capital Gaborone, situated in the southeast at 3,215 feet (979.9 meters) elevation with a population of nearly 250,000.[2] Gaborone is pronounced "ha-bo-ro-neh," but locals often refer to it as "Gabs." Gaborone is host to the headquarters of the Southern African Development Community—a regionally vital fifteen-nation intergovernmental organization which is dedicated to socioeconomic, political, and security cooperation in southern Africa, but is hardly known in nonpolitical U.S. circles. The second largest city is Francistown, north of the Tropic of Capricorn. Most of the population lives in Gaborone and Francistown and in the southeast of the country.

Brief History of Botswana

In the nineteenth century there were escalating tensions in what is now Botswana among the Tswana and Ndebele tribes and the Boer settlers who had migrated north from the Transvaal (now part of South Africa). In March 1885, after appeals by the Batswana, (a term used to refer to all indigenous tribes) leaders, the British government put Bechuanaland (a land greater in size than current Botswana) under its protection. The north remained under British administration as the Bechuanaland Protectorate, and in June 1964 became Botswana. The south eventually became part of South Africa.

In 1965, the capital was established in Gaborone. In 1966, independence was declared, and Seretse Khama was elected as the first president. Sir Seretse Khama is regarded as a hero in Botswana, and his name can be found on many landmarks, such as the airport. He was educated in South Africa and at Oxford University, became president, was reelected twice, and died in office in 1980. Under Khama the country made tremendous economic and social progress. Khama forced an early reckoning with race relations in the country by his marriage to a white woman, Ruth Williams.

The Botswana presidency has changed hands relatively few times. After Sir Seretse Khama died, the presidency passed to the vice president, Ouett Masire, who was then elected in 1984, 1989, and 1994. Masire retired in 1998. His vice president, Festus Mogae, became president in 1999 and was reelected in 2004. The current president is Lieutenant General Seretse Khama Ian Khama, the eldest son of Sir Seretse Khama.

The People and Culture

The Botswana population is estimated at 1,990,876.[3] The population density is extremely low, less than three people per square kilometer (or fewer than three per ⅞ square mile), and the estimated annual population growth rate is 1.937 percent.[4] Currently, life expectancy in Botswana is fifty-one years on average (51 years for males and fifty-two years for females), a tragic fall from the pre-HIV epidemic life expectancy of sixty-five.[5]

English is the official language and Setswana is the most commonly spoken national language. Most educated residents of Gabarone speak English, but patients from remote areas who are seen in the national health service system may not. *Setswana* is not only a language but is also used as the adjective to describe the cultural traditions of the Batswana, the indigenous people of Botswana.[6] It is also an appropriate way to refer to the people of Botswana (plural *Setswana*, singular *Motswana*). Christianity is by far the most common religion in Botswana, followed by Badimo (a traditional religion in Botswana in which ancestors are believed to play a significant role in daily life), Islam, and Hindu, but many people still practice traditional animist beliefs.

For travelers going to visit Botswana, there are many sources for appropriate cultural adaptation.[7] One important cultural concept for visitors engaging in healthcare program development and research to understand is that of the *kgotla* (pronounced "hoat-la"). A *kgotla* is a public meeting, community council, or traditional law court in which community decisions are arrived at by consensus. It is vital to note that anyone is allowed to speak, and no one may interrupt while someone is having their say. The custom of allowing everyone their full say is relevant in meetings of all kinds, such as staff meetings, and can result in meetings lasting many hours.

Literature

Botswana has a rich literary culture. Bessie Head is usually considered Botswana's most important writer. She fled the apartheid regime in South Africa to live in and write about Botswana until her death at the age of forty-nine in 1986. She lived in the small Botswana city of Serowe, and her most famous books are set there, including *When Rain Clouds Gather*, *Maru*, and *A Question of Power*.

Botswana is also the setting for the currently extremely successful series of mystery novels by Alexander McCall Smith,[8] the first of which is called *The No. 1 Ladies' Detective Agency*. The series has now been adapted for television (BBC and HBO) and radio (BBC). The series' protagonist, Precious Ramotswe, lives in Gaborone. The books are a should-read as an insight into local settings and culture.

Other noteworthy authors include Norman Rush, who served as Peace Corps director in Botswana from 1978 to 1983. He uses Botswana as the setting of his novels and book of short stories which generally focus on the expatriate community. Unity Dow came from a rural setting in which her mother could not read English, and where in most cases, decision making was done by men. She became a lawyer, human rights activist, and the country's first female High Court judge. Her four books are concerned with the struggle between Western and traditional values, gender issues and poverty: *Far and Beyon', The Screaming of the Innocent, Juggling Truth*, and *The Heavens May Fall*. Mark and Delia Owens chronicled their remarkable wildlife adventure of self-isolation in the harshest of Botswana terrains in the best-selling book *Cry of the Kalahari*. The Owens went on to successfully advocate for preservation of the Kalahari Desert.

Botswana was also the location for the 1980 movie *The Gods Must Be Crazy*, by Jamie Uys. In this cult classic, a Sho of the Kalahari first encounters Western culture in the form of a Coke bottle discarded from a passing plane.

Economy and Income

Since independence in September 1966, Botswana has had one of the fastest growth rates in per capita income in the world. It is considered a middle-income country, with a per capita gross domestic product (GDP; see the glossary) of $14,100 in 2008. Economic growth averaged over 9 percent per year from 1967 to 2006, but has fallen since to approximately 5% in 2009, as economic development spending was reduced, in part as a result of rising expenditure on healthcare services due to the AIDS epidemic. Botswana's currency, the *pula* (which is also the Setswana word for rain), is valued against currencies heavily weighted toward the South African Rand.

Diamonds are Botswana's chief national export. Diamond mining accounts for more than one-third of GDP and for 70 to 80 percent of export earnings; Botswana's economic growth and success has been built on the foundation of using the revenue generated from diamond mining to fuel its economic development. Debswana, the largest diamond mining company, is an important national presence. Debswana is 50 percent government owned and generates about half of all government revenues.

Education and Literacy

Botswana has a high literacy rate (81.2 percent),[9] and the net enrollment rate in primary education is 84.1 percent.[10] In Botswana's education system, girls and boys have equal access to education. Girls, however, have a high likelihood of dropping out of secondary school due to pregnancy.

All students are guaranteed ten years of basic education, leading to a Junior Certificate qualification. Approximately half of the school population attends a further two years of secondary schooling, leading to the Botswana General Certificate of Secondary Education. After leaving school, students can attend one of the six technical colleges in the country or take vocational training courses in teaching or nursing. The best students enter the University of Botswana in Gaborone, a modern, well-resourced campus with a student population of over ten thousand.

Unfortunately, in January 2006, the government of Botswana reintroduced school fees, which may serve as a deterrent to education for the poorest children. The government still provides full funding to any Motswana attending the University of Botswana or a university abroad if the appropriate education is not offered locally, such as medicine. Of note, a Botswana medical school appears imminent and is in formation with leadership from Baylor College of Medicine, in Houston, Texas.

The Healthcare System in Botswana

The healthcare delivery system of Botswana is based on the principles of a primary healthcare model with integrated service delivery at the local level.[11] The country is divided into twenty-four health districts (which can be confusing because recall that the country is made up of nine government administrative districts). The government, through the Ministry of Health (MOH), is the principal healthcare provider. The MOH is responsible for the national health, including policies, goals, and strategies for health development and delivery. The district and local authorities are responsible for delivery of primary healthcare services through health posts, which serve remote and rural areas, clinics, primary hospitals, and district hospitals. The central government provides referral services at Princess Marina Hospital in Gaborone and Francistown Hospital in Francistown. Hospital care, medications, and laboratory tests are free for all citizens in public-sector facilities.

Hospitals and the twenty-four local health districts administer local clinics. Each district has a district health team led by a public health specialist who is responsible for administration and supervision of a number of public health–oriented services, such as tuberculosis (TB) and HIV. In addition to government-sponsored institutions, faith-based organizations (FBOS; see the glossary), other nongovernmental organizations (NGOS; see the glossary), and mining companies provide a parallel system of private healthcare through a complementary network of hospitals and clinics.[12]

Leading Health Issues in Botswana

HIV/AIDS

Botswana is experiencing one of the most severe HIV/AIDS epidemics in the world. The national HIV prevalence rate (see the glossary) among adults ages fifteen to forty-nine is 23.9 percent, which is second only to Swaziland.[13] The primary mode of transmission is heterosexual contact. The prevalence of HIV is higher in women than in men. For example, young women ages fifteen to twenty-four have an HIV prevalence rate of 15.3 percent, while young men in the same age group experience prevalence rates of 5.1 percent.[14] HIV infection rates vary by geographical region and are highest in towns, lower in cities, and lowest in villages. The United Nations Development Programme estimates that at least 20 percent of all children in Botswana are orphans, and seventy-six percent of the country's orphaned children have lost their parents to AIDS.[15] A useful history of the incredible story of HIV/AIDS in Botswana, including an overview of current HIV prevention, testing and treatment strategies, is provided at the website of AVERT, an international AIDS charity.[16]

In response to these staggering statistics, the government of Botswana has developed one of Africa's most comprehensive programs of HIV/AIDS prevention, treatment, and care. Botswana's first AIDS case was reported in 1985. From 1987 through 1989, Botswana's response to HIV/AIDS focused mainly on screening blood to eliminate the risk of HIV transmission through blood transfusion. From 1989 through 1997, the government's first Medium Term Plan introduced information, education, and communication programs, and in 1993 the Botswana National Policy on AIDS was adopted.[17] Since 1997 additional prevention efforts and comprehensive care have been implemented, including the provision of antiretroviral therapy (ART; see the glossary). The second Medium Term Plan (1997–2002) was developed with the overall goal of continuing to reduce HIV transmission and to mitigate the national impact of HIV/AIDS.[18]

Voluntary HIV counseling and testing (VCT) has been essential to HIV prevention and care.[19] Since 2000, the government of Botswana and the U.S. Centers for Disease Control and Prevention (CDC), through BOTUSA (Bostwana-USA, described in detail later in this chapter), have developed and supported the extensive Tebelopele network of VCT centers which provide immediate, free, confidential VCT services for Batswana. Although originally connected to BOTUSA, Tebelopele became an independent NGO in 2004.

The Tebelopele network has been an international model of VCT, including its successful marketing campaign—"Know Your Status" and "Show You Care"—developed by the CDC in collaboration with Population Services International. These campaigns have been promoted through an unprecedented number of billboards, banners, and other print messages; advertisements at bus stops; and regular radio programs throughout Botswana.

In 1999, the National AIDS Coordinating Agency was formed and made responsible for mobilizing and coordinating a multi-sectoral national response to HIV and AIDS. The agency works under the National AIDS Council, which is chaired by the president of Botswana and has representatives from seventeen agencies and organizations, including civil societies (NGOS), the public sector and the private sector.

The country's ART program has also been a model of AIDS care in Africa. The national ART program was given the name *MASA*, the Setswana world for dawn. In January 2002, antiretrovirals were first made available through the public sector at the Princess Marina Hospital in Gaborone. By the end of 2006, some 84,000 people were receiving treatment, a number that exceeded 95 percent of the population in need.[20]

Tuberculosis

Botswana also has one of the highest rates of TB (see the glossary) in the world, with 731 cases per 100,000 population in 2007 (the year with most complete current data).[21] This translates to nearly 14,000 cases in the country in 2007. The overall mortality rate of TB is 37/100,000 population. The TB mortality rate is higher among HIV-infected persons, at 157/100,000. Indeed, TB is the leading cause of death for HIV-infected persons in Africa.

To control TB, the Botswana National Tuberculosis Programme was established in 1975, with technical assistance from the World Health Organization (WHO). The programme (which is part of the Disease Control Unit within the Health Ministry's Department of Public Health) introduced the recommended short course chemotherapy for treatment of TB in 1986, and adopted WHO's full directly observed therapy (DOTS; see the glossary) TB control strategy in 1993. In 2007, there was 100 percent DOTS coverage in Botswana.[22]

One public health specialist, one senior medical officer and two technical officers currently staff the National Tuberculosis Programme. There are also three principal health officers and two data entry clerks who were recruited for implementation of the National Isoniazid Preventive Therapy (IPT) Programme. The day-to-day coordination of the program's activities is the responsibility of the district TB coordinators. Twenty of the twenty-four health districts have no full-time district TB coordinators at the time of this writing.

The high rate of TB in Botswana is largely attributable to the HIV epidemic, since HIV makes persons more susceptible to TB, and there is more subsequent TB transmission in communities both to HIV-infected and to uninfected persons. In 2007, 68 percent of the TB patients in Botswana who were tested were HIV-infected, and we have observed an even higher proportion among those TB patients who require hospitalization.[23]

One major and noteworthy effort to control TB among HIV-infected persons in Botswana has been that of the isoniazid preventive therapy (IPT) program. Isoniazid therapy does prevent the development of TB in HIV-infected persons, and in 1998, the Joint WHO/UN Guidelines on HIV/AIDS recommended the use of IPT in HIV-TB co-epidemic settings. In 1999, the Botswana government formed the IPT Working Group, which by 2000 had begun a pilot program of IPT administration in three healthdistricts. The pilot program was completed, evaluated, and deemed successful enough to warrant national rollout through integration into general clinical services, which was completed by 2004. Botswana has therefore been a model for IPT administration in Africa.[24]

On a more sobering note, TB that is resistant to standard or first-line drug treatment has been identified in Botswana. Over 100 people have been diagnosed with multidrug-resistant TB (MDR TB; see the glossary) in Botswana. In 2007, 0.8 percent of patients presenting for TB treatment for the first time and 10 percent of those presenting for retreatment had MDR TB.[25] The government of Botswana announced recently that two cases of extensively drug-resistant tuberculosis (XDR TB; see the glossary) have been identified.[26] They are the first cases to be reported in sub-Saharan Africa outside South Africa. XDR TB is very difficult and costly to treat, and it may have increased mortality in people with HIV. It can be diagnosed only by laboratories equipped to carry out drug susceptibility testing, so its prevalence in sub-Saharan Africa is not yet known. Nearly 500 cases of XDR TB have been diagnosed in South Africa since 2006, when an outbreak was first identified in KwaZulu Natal province.[27]

Health Agencies and Their Initiatives in Botswana

The most significant partners with the Botswana government for AIDS initiatives are the African Comprehensive HIV/AIDS Partnerships (ACHAP), the Botswana Christian AIDS Intervention Program (BOCAIP), the BOTUSA Project, the Global Fund to Fight AIDS, Tuberculosis and Malaria (see the glossary), the Harvard School of Public Health, the Bristol-Myers Squibb Foundation, the University of Pennsylvania, and numerous faith-based and community-based organizations, all described below.

The African Comprehensive HIV/AIDS Partnerships (ACHAP) was established in July 2000 for HIV/AIDS response. It is an important collaboration between the government of Botswana, the Bill & Melinda Gates Foundation, and the Merck Company Foundation. The Bill & Melinda Gates Foundation and the Merck Company Foundation each committed $50 million to the project, and Merck also donated supplies of two antiretroviral drugs for use in the public sector.

The Botswana Christian AIDS Intervention Program (BOCAIP) is an NGO of Christians against AIDS in Botswana, founded in 1996. BOCAIP draws Christian membership from the academic sector, other parts of the private sector, and the government. Significant funding is provided by Bristol-Myers Squibb's "Secure the Future" project and ACHAP. ACHAP and BOCAIP collaborated to establish eleven HIV/AIDS counseling centers. These centers train many counselors and provide services to persons living with HIV/AIDS.

In 1995, the CDC and the Botswana government began a collaboration called BOTUSA, which "provides training, technical assistance and research; promotes innovation and evidence-based best practices; and supports the monitoring and evaluation of prevention, care and treatment programs for HIV/AIDS and TB."[28] BOTUSA is closely linked to the CDC's Global AIDS Program and the President's Emergency Plan for AIDS Relief (PEPFAR; see the glossary), which provides substantial financial support to HIV/AIDS programs in Botswana — $93.2 million in fiscal year 2008, and $93.9 million planned for FY 2009.[29] In response to the shortage of human resources for provision of antiretrovirals, the Harvard AIDS Initiative and the Botswana Ministry of Health established the KITSO (Knowledge, Innovation and Training Shall Overcome AIDS) Training Program in 2000, to provide training in HIV and AIDS care for Botswana's health professionals. Support for KITSO is also provided by ACHAP.

Since 1999, through the company's Secure the Future Program, Bristol-Myers Squibb and the Bristol-Myers Squibb Foundation have committed $150 million to develop solutions for vulnerable populations, including women and children, infected and affected by HIV/AIDS in twelve countries in sub-Saharan Africa, including Botswana.[30]

The government of Botswana, ACHAP, the University of Botswana and the University of Pennsylvania formed the Botswana-UPenn Partnership to build HIV/AIDS expertise in Botswana in response to the HIV/AIDS epidemic. UPenn helps train local healthcare providers in the prevention and treatment of HIV/AIDS and its complications, develops postgraduate training programs at the University of Botswana, and develops joint research programs. Students from the University of Pennsylvania also come to Botswana for global health training.

Other Issues of Interest in Botswana

Bushmen

The San, Sho, Basarwa, Kung, and Khwe tribes constitute the Bushmen, indigenous people of southern Africa. Botswana has the largest population of these First Nation People: 55,000 of the estimated 90,000 indigenous people of southern Africa reside in Botswana. Batswana most commonly refer to these people as *Basarwa*, which is a largely pejorative term. They were traditionally hunter-gatherers in the Central Kalahari Game Reserve. In the mid-1990s, the government of Botswana attempted to force them to switch to farming as part of a policy to relocate them to newly created settlements off the reserve. The government denied that the relocation had been forced, but on December 13, 2006, a court ruling confirmed that the removal was forced and unconstitutional.[31] In spite of the ruling, only a limited number of Bushmen have been allowed to return to the Central Kalahari Game Reserve.

Conflict Diamonds

A conflict diamond (also called a converted diamond, blood diamond, hot diamond, or war diamond) refers to a diamond that was mined in an area controlled by forces opposed to legitimate and internationally recognized governments, and whose mining is used to fund military action in opposition to those governments.[32] There is increasing attention to stemming the traffic in conflict diamonds, which may decrease the overall diamond market. In popular culture, the movie *Blood Diamond*—starring Leonardo DiCaprio, Jennifer Connelly, and Djimon Hounsou—has highlighted this issue. Although Botswana's diamond exports are certified according to international standards as nonconflict, if the great demand for diamonds were to decline the economy of Botswana would suffer greatly, as the country is highly dependent on this export.

Advice for Travelers to Botswana

The U.S. State Department has vital information for anyone traveling to Botswana.[33] A passport with at least six months of validity remaining is required. At the time of this writing, U.S. citizens are permitted stays up to ninety days without a visa, but for the most up-to-date information on entry requirements, travelers should contact the Embassy of the Republic of Botswana in Washington, D.C., or the Permanent Mission of the Republic of Botswana to the United Nations in New York City. Of note, visitors to Botswana who intend to visit South Africa, as well, should know that their passport must contain at least two blank (unstamped) visa pages each time entry to South Africa is sought. Otherwise, you may be refused entry into South Africa, fined, and returned to your point of origin within Africa at your own expense.

Civil unrest is unusual in Botswana, and overall the crime rate is similar to that of any large urban area. Pedestrians are advised to avoid walking in Gaborone and other urban areas in Botswana at night. The Caprivi Strip, a narrow strip of land belonging to Namibia and bordering northwest Botswana, is unstable because of armed rebel activity by a rebel group seeking secession of the region from Namibia, and the U.S. State Department recommends that U.S. citizens do not travel the Trans Caprivi Highway at night.

Most travelers arriving in Botswana do so via South Africa. Travelers should be aware that there is often theft from baggage in transit at Johannesburg and Cape Town international airports. You should never place any valuables in checked luggage.

Driving in Botswana is challenging and high risk. Traffic circulates on the left in Botswana. While the roads in major population centers are generally good, many roads are vulnerable to damage by heavy summer rains.

The U.S. Department of State considers "medical facilities in Gaborone adequate for simple medical problems, but facilities outside of Gaborone are limited."[34] Professional private emergency rescue services operate air and ground ambulances throughout the country, but care is rendered only after a patient's ability to pay is established. Therefore, having adequate evacuation coverage is a high priority. For advanced medical care, Americans often choose to travel to South Africa (Pretoria, for example).

Conclusion

The general consensus is that Botswana is a wonderful place to work. In broad strokes, it is beautiful, relatively safe and stable, with more resources than most African countries, and is a place where one can work effectively with local collaborators. Gaborone itself is a small and manageable city, with a public transport service, access to high-quality goods, unique crafts, a few gyms, and some entertainment in the form of cultural live music and movie theaters.

A few insider tips may help smooth your transition into the Botswana culture. Because there are many NGOs and expatriates in Gaborone, most Batswana in the city are used to working with Americans. The style of meetings, processes, and hierarchies may appear very American. However, there are important differences. For example, as described in chapter 2, it may not be possible to accomplish your goals at the same pace that you are used to at home. We observed a common affliction in the medical students coming to work with us: "deceleration injuries" were frequent among those coming fresh from intense, busy rotations to a setting where meetings may not happen on time, navigating the required procedures, protocols, and business etiquette is time consuming, and the *kgotla* principle is operative: everyone gets a say. In addition, if you want your project to be successful, you must work within the hierarchy and make sure that everyone is included. Even if you have permission for activities from a person in authority, it will be worthwhile to inquire if there is anyone else to brief and include. The answer is usually yes. Your local colleagues will help you navigate this.

Batswana are friendly but proud people. There are topics best not talked about except in the most intimate friendships. It is famously inappropriate to ask Batswana how many cows they have, since this is a certain measure of wealth and akin to asking how much one has in their bank account. Always bear in mind that there are significant disparities in resources between you and most of your counterparts: don't flaunt your relative wealth. It is okay to ask about which village someone comes from, but may not be appropriate to inquire to which tribe a Motswana belongs.

Fascinating and sometimes difficult differences exist between perceptions of sexuality and gender roles. A majority of Batswana—men and women alike—endorse the saying, "A man like a bull should not be confined to one pasture." As in other places in Africa, women are more subject to the authority of their partner (or husband), and more likely subject to physical abuse than are men.

A very simple cultural mistake to avoid is based on the typical observation that professional dress is more formal in Botswana. Despite sometimes very hot conditions, you should be prepared to wear a shirt and tie or skirt or dress for all professional gatherings. This concept is described in more detail in chapter 2. Remember, too, that the winter is actually cold—nothing says unprepared more than coming with a suitcase of T-shirts and shorts to work in August.

Despite many Batswana's extensive collaborations with Americans, be aware that people initially may be wary of you and your work. Avoid at all costs any project that can be construed or wind up as "data rape" — a foreign researcher who swoops in for a short time, takes valuable data, and then returns to the United States to publish it and catapult his or her own career, never providing final reports, co-authorship, or follow up to local collaborators. However, we trust once you take time to get to know your collaborators, the basics of the culture, and this wonderful country, this would seem outrageous behavior.

Enjoy your time in beautiful Botswana. As we have attempted to describe, it is a setting remarkable for many reasons: stunning wild spaces, tremendous public health challenges, and a team of nationals and expatriates committed to overcoming these challenges. For such a small country, Botswana makes a big and lasting impression on everyone from international health policymakers to the short-term student tourist. With preparation and an open mind and heart, the lessons learned in Botswana can launch and inform a successful career in global health.

COUNTRY DATA : BOTSWANA

Millennium Development Goal indicators are italicized.

TABLE 3.1 : POPULATION AND HUMAN DEVELOPMENT

POPULATION

Total	1.99 million
Population growth rate	1.94%
Net migration rate/1,000 population	5.0
Urban	60.0%
Rural	40.0%

AGE STRUCTURE

0–14 years	34.8%
15–64 years	61.4%
65+ years	3.8%
Median age (years)	21.7

MAJOR ETHNIC GROUPS

Tswana	79%
Kalanga	11%
Basarwa	3%
Other, including Kgalagadi and White	7%

RELIGIONS

Christian	60%
Badimo	6%
Islam	1%
Hindu	< 1%
None	20%

HUMAN DEVELOPMENT

Human Development Index	0.664
Human Development rank[a]	126th
Freedom House Index	Free
Political Rights score[b]	2
Civil Liberties score[b]	2
Human Poverty Index	31.4%
Human Poverty rank[c]	124th

Notes: [a]out of 179 countries; [b]1 = most free, 7 = least free; [c]out of 177 countries

TABLE 3.2 : **GOVERNMENT AND ECONOMY**

GOVERNMENT	
Independence	30 Sep.1966 from Britain
Type of government	Parliamentary republic
Voting rights	Age 18, universal
CAPITAL	Gaborone
CURRENCY	Pula (BWP)
ECONOMY	
Gross domestic product (GDP) (in PPP US $)	267.06 billion
Annual GDP growth	5.0%
GDP per capita (in US $)	$14,100
Gini Index	63
Population living below PPP $1/day	*31.2%*
Public debt as % of GDP	5.9
Official development assistance (ODA) per capita (in US $)	$40.2
Foreign direct investment as % of GDP	2.7
LABOR FORCE	
In agriculture	NA
In industry	NA
In services	NA
Unemployment rate	7.5%

TABLE 3.3 : GEOGRAPHY AND ENVIRONMENT

LAND COMPOSITION

Land area	581,730 sq. km. (224,607 sq. mi.)
Size comparison	Slightly smaller than Texas
Terrain	Flat or gently rolling tableland; Kalahari Desert in southwest; landlocked
Ecological hazards	Droughts, August winds carrying sand and dust

LAND USE AND RESOURCES

Permanent crop land	0.01%
Arable land	0.65%
Agricultural products	Livestock, sorghum, maize, millet, beans, sunflowers
Natural resources	Diamonds, copper, nickel, salt, soda ash, potash, coal, iron ore, silver

ENVIRONMENTAL ISSUES	Overgrazing, desertification, limited fresh water resources

INFRASTRUCTURE

Population with access to improved water source	96%
Population using improved sanitation	47%
Roadways unpaved	67.4%

TABLE 3.4 : HEALTH

LIFE, BIRTH, DEATH

Life expectancy at birth (male/female)	51/52
Birth rate/1,000 population	22.89
Death rate/1,000 population	8.52
Infant mortality rate/1,000 live births	*33.0*

PERSONNEL AND INFRASTRUCTURE

Physicians/100,000 population	40
Hospital beds/10,000 population	24

HEALTH ECONOMICS

Total expenditure on health per capita (PPP US $)	$504
Public expenditure on health as % of GDP	4.0

Most common vector-borne disease	Malaria
Most common food- and water-borne diseases	Bacterial diarrhea, hepatitis A, typhoid fever
TB incidence/100,000 population	*731.4*
TB prevalence/100,000 population	*622.2*
New TB cases HIV-positive	68%
New TB cases multidrug-resistant (MDR)	0.8%
1-year-olds fully immunized against TB	99%
Estimated malaria cases annually	NA
Malaria death rate/100,000 population	NA
HIV prevalence rate in adults	*23.9%*
AIDS deaths in adults annually	*11,000*
People living with HIV	300,000
AIDS orphans	95,000

MATERNAL HEALTH

Fertility rate (children born per woman)	2.66
Contraceptive prevalence rate (married women 15–49)	*48%*
Maternal mortality rate/100,000 births	*380*
Lifetime risk of maternal death, 1 in:	*130*
Births attended by skilled birth attendant	*94%*

CHILD HEALTH

Mortality rate of children < 5/1,000 live births	*40*
1-year-olds immunized against measles	*90%*
Children < 5 using insecticide-treated bed nets	*< 10%*
Children < 5 with fever treated with antimalarial drugs	*NA*
Newborns protected against tetanus	78%

HUNGER AND MALNUTRITION

Children < 5 underweight for age	*14%*
Children < 5 under height for age	*29%*
Population undernourished	*26%*

TABLE 3.5 : LANGUAGE, EDUCATION, AND LITERACY

LANGUAGES	
Setswana	78%
Kalanga	8%
Sekgalagdi	3%
English (official language)	2%
Other	9%
LITERACY	
Adult literacy rate (population age 15+ who can read and write)	81.2%
EXPENDITURE	
Public expenditure on education as % of GDP	8.7
EDUCATION	
Primary mandatory	Yes
Secondary mandatory	No
Net enrollment in primary education[d]	*84.1%*
School life expectancy, in years (male/female)[e]	12/12

[d]Net enrollment rate in primary education is measured as the number of children of official primary school age who are enrolled in primary education as a percentage of children in the official primary school age population.

[e]School life expectancy is the total number of years of school (from primary through tertiary education) that a child can expect to receive.

Principal Sources for Data in Appendix Tables 3.1–3.5

Central Intelligence Agency, *The World Factbook* (https://www.cia.gov/library/publications/the-world-factbook/).

UN Millennium Development Goals Indicators Database (http://millenniumindicators.un.org/unsd/mdg/).

UNDP Human Development Report, 2007/2008 (http://hdr.undp.org/en/reports/global/hdr2007-2008/).

UNICEF. The State of the World's Children 2009 (http://www.unicef.org/publications/index_47127.html).

NOTES

1. Central Intelligence Agency, The World Factbook, Botswana (https://www.cia.gov/library/publication/the-world-factbook/geos/bc.html).

2. Botswana Export Development and Investment Authority, BEDIA. (http://www.bedia.co.bw/article.php?id_mnu=37).

3. Central Intelligence Agency, The World Factbook. Botswana.

4. Ibid.

5. World Health Organization, Botswana (http://www.who.int/countries/bwa/en).

6. All indigenous people of Botswana are commonly known as Batswana (plural, with singular being Motswana.) In the Setswana language the names of all indigenous tribes have the prefix "Ba" added before the word, for instance, Bamangwaro, Batawana, etc.

7. See, for instance, Michael Main, *Botswana—Culture Smart!* with a quick guide to customs and etiquette (London: Kuperard, 2007).

8. See his website at http://www.randomhouse.com/features/mccallsmith/main.php.

9. Central Intelligence Agency, The World Factbook, Botswana.

10. Net enrollment rate in primary education is a Millennium Development Goal indicator. It is measured as the number of children of primary school age who are enrolled in primary education in the country as a percentage of children in the primary school age population; United Nations Children's Fund, "The State of the World's Children." UNdata. Net enrollment/attendance rate in primary education, 2010 (http://data.un.org/Data.aspx?d=SOWC&f=inID%3A129).

11. The website of Botswana's Ministry of Health allows you to explore the structure of health care delivery and all functions carried out by the Ministry. See (http://www.moh.gov.bw/index.php?option=com_content1&id=1).

12. Ibid.

13. United Nations Children's Fund, "The State of the World's Children." UNdata, Adult HIV/AIDS Prevalence Rate, 2010. (http://data.un.org/Data.aspx?q=hIV+prevalence+rate&d=SOWC&f=inID%3a73)

14. Ibid.

15. AVERT, "AIDS orphans" (http://www.avert.org/aids-orphans.htm).

16. AVERT, "HIV & AIDS in Botswana." (http://www.avert.org/aids-botswana.htm).

17. See "History of HIV and AIDS in Botswana," at www.avert.org/aidsbotswana.htm.

18. Ibid.

19. T. L. Creek, et al., "Botswana's Tebelopele Voluntary Counseling and Testing Network: Use and Client Risk Factors for HIV Infection, 2000-2004," *Journal of Acquired Immune Deficiency Syndromes* 43, no. 2 (2006): 210-18.

20. World Health Organization, "Towards Universal Access: Scaling Up Priority HIV/AIDS Interventions in the Health Sector." (Geneva: WHO, September 2009; http://www.who.int/hiv/pub/2009progressreport/en/index.html).

21. World Health Organization, "Global Tuberculosis Control: WHO Report

2009." Africa. (http://www.who.int/tb/publications/global_report/2009/pdf/annex3_afr.pdf).

22. Ibid.

23. Elizabeth A. Talbot et al., "Tuberculosis Serodiagnosis in a Predominantly HIV-infected Population of Hospitalized Patients with Cough, Botswana, 2002" *Clinical Infectious Diseases* 39, no. 1 (2004): e1–7.

24. Aidsmap, "IPT: barriers to national implementation" 29 November 2007 (http://www.aidsmap.com/resources/hatip/IPT-barriers-to-national-implementation/page/1255942/); B. Mosimaneotsile et al., "Value of Chest Radiography in a Tuberculosis Prevention Programme for HIV-infected People, Botswana," *Lancet* 362, no. 9395 (2003): 1551–52.

25. World Health Organization, "Global Tuberculosis Control: WHO Report 2009."

26. Keith Alcorn. "Two XDR TB cases reported in Botswana," aidsmap, 17 January 2008 (http://www.aidsmap.com/en/Email-a-friend/tpl/1412195/page/1429259/).

27. This outbreak is described in detail in the South Africa chapter.

28. Centers for Disease Control and Prevention, "BOTUSA: A United States Botswana Partnership" (http://www.cdc.gov/botusa/).

29. The United States President's Emergency Plan for AIDS Relief, "Partnership to Fight HIV/AIDS in Botswana" (http://www.pepfar.gov/countries/botswana/index.htm).

30. Bristol-Myers Squibb, "Secure the Future" (http://www.securethefuture.com/).

31. Kgeikani Kweni, First People of the Kalahari, "I want 2 go home" (http://www.iwant2gohome.org), and Carolyn Dempster, "Botswana Bushmen's last stand," BBC News, 18 March 2002 (http://news.bbc.uk/2/hi/africa/1879429.stm).

32. United Nations Department of Public Information, "Conflict Diamonds" (21 March 2001 http://www.un.org/peace/africa/Diamond.html).

33. See the U.S. Department of State's website (http://travel.state.gov/travel/cis_pa_tw/cis/cis_1071.html).

34. Ibid.

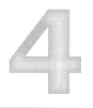

JOYCE A. SACKEY

NAMEETA M. DOOKERAN

STELLA SAFO

GHANA

Ghana has enjoyed relative stability since this West African country first became independent in 1957. This geopolitical stability, coupled with a rich history and a reputation as a friendly nation, make Ghana a favorite destination for volunteer groups and global health workers. Many international agencies and nongovernmental organizations (NGOS; see the glossary) have offices and a sizable presence of aid workers in the country. Ghana enjoys the distinction of being the first country in the world to accept Peace Corp volunteers, and its program has remained one of the largest. Over the decades, U.S. volunteers have been involved with programs in education, agriculture, business, health, water sanitation, and youth empowerment and education. Many U.S.-based schools and universities have established exchanges with counterpart institutions in Ghana, so students at all levels of training participate in study abroad or exchange programs in the country. In addition, a growing number of churches from around the world have established regular medical missions to Ghana, typically in collaboration with "sister" churches in Ghana. These medical missions offer their congregants the opportunity to make a difference through volunteerism. Not surprisingly, then, there is a growing demand for practical resources that can serve as part of an orientation for the health worker preparing to go to Ghana.

This chapter provides a brief history of Ghana from its earliest days of settlement, to the colonial era when Ghana was referred to as the Gold Coast, and its struggle for independence. Then we discuss current geopolitical and socioeconomic trends in the country, its educational and health systems, and important cultural, health, and other contextual considerations that should inform the work of any health professional or volunteer seeking to successfully implement a community development project, engage in research, or provide direct patient care in Ghana.

History and Geography

Ghana is a small nation (239,460 square kilometers, or 92,456 square miles) in West Africa, surrounded in the south by the Atlantic Ocean and in the north, east, and west by the Francophone countries of Burkina Faso, Togo, and the Côte d'Ivoire, respectively. Ghana's three ecological zones — savannas, coastal lands, and tropical rainforests — and alternating wet and dry seasonal changes have made it both rich in natural resources, like cocoa and gold, and replete with such tropical diseases as yellow fever and malaria.

Present-day Ghana was settled by hunter-gatherer groups as far back as the Stone Age, some 50,000 years ago. The ancestors of contemporary ethnic groups such as the Akan and the Ga-Dangme began settling in the region around 2000 BCE. Early archaeological records show that many of these groups emigrated from surrounding West African territories — the current countries of Nigeria, Togo, and Benin. Once settled, pre-colonial Ghana flourished as several autonomous and often conflicting tribal nations. The northern ethnic groups were the first to form centralized states in the seventeenth century under Islamic rule. The south, home to the Akan ethnic group, was ruled by the powerful Asante tribe that wielded political and military power over the region through the formation of the Asante Confederacy in the eighteenth century. The tenuous balance of power shared by Ghana's pre-colonial ethnic states would be greatly disturbed by the entrance of Europeans in the fifteenth century.

Ghana's natural resources and its coastal location made it a long-coveted prize during the centuries of European exploration and colonization of the African mainland. The Portuguese were the first Europeans to settle along Ghana's coast, in 1471. They built coastal forts, as did the Dutch who came to Ghana in the late sixteenth century. These early forts would become the slave castles from which human, manufactured, and natural resources from the heartland of Africa were shipped to other parts of the world.

However, it was the British who had the most lasting impact. British merchants could be found in Ghana as early as 1631. Like other Europeans, the British settled along the coast and accessed Ghana's wealth of natural resources by interfacing with the chiefs and traditional leaders of local tribes. Since the Asante were the most powerful ethnic group, the British were forced to abide by their rules and whims in order to gain access to important trade routes and resources. It was not long before British merchants realized that they could have greater control over the area and its resources if they could end the Asante's regional dominance.

With destabilization of the Asante kingdom as the ultimate goal, the British and a few local tribes hoping to gain from an alliance with the Europeans waged the 1874 Sagrenti War. Despite the best efforts of the Asante warriors, the British defeated them. The symbol of sovereignty of the *Asantehene* (the Asante king) and hence the entire Asante kingdom and culture was a golden stool, thought to contain the soul of the Asante nation and considered sacred. The British worked tirelessly to obtain the golden stool as a sign of their new acquisition of power. Although they failed to gain possession of the golden stool, the British declared control over the region in 1874. They drew the lands of the north, the central Asante area, and the coastal trading grounds under one title: the Colony of the Gold Coast. A final battle was fought in 1901, when remaining Asante leaders attempted to regain control. A second British victory led to the Gold Coast's becoming a colony under full British governance.

Ghana's colonial period was marked by rapid expansion of production and economic growth. The export of goods to England fueled all aspects of the colony's activities. Not surprisingly, there were growing conflicts between the indigenous population and British nationals, particularly over the distribution of land. These sentiments worsened after World War II, when some of the 70,000 Ghanaian solders who had fought alongside the British for the freedom of other nations returned home to question their country's status as a colony. A strong and growing nationalistic sentiment led to the creation of the United Gold Coast Convention in 1947, whose goal was to obtain self-governance within the shortest period of time. In 1949, the Convention People's Party—with its slogan "self-government now," its more aggressive advance of the aim of independence, and its charismatic leader Kwame Nkrumah—

laid the foundation for the end of British rule. With careful diplomacy by its leaders and concerted pressure from the populace, Ghana became the first West African nation to gain independence, on March 6, 1957, under Nkrumah's leadership. Nkrumah's pan-African vision led him to help foster other African countries to gain their own independence.

Ghana's first years following independence were marked by notable achievements and some remarkable technological advances for the region, including the construction of the Akosombo Dam, and the establishment of one of the first African international airlines and shipping companies, Ghana Airways and Black Star Shipping Lines.

However, the new nation's initial success was followed by years of political upheaval; a series of military coups replaced democratically elected governments, forcing the country through economic and civil hardship. In 1966, a combined military and police force under Lieutenant General Joseph Ankrah overthrew Nkrumah's government and established the National Liberation Council. The council facilitated democratic elections in 1969, and K. A. Busia was chosen as prime minister to head the government. In 1972, Busia's Progress Party was overthrown by Colonel I. K. Acheampong's army, which in turn established the National Redemption Council. This group attempted to return the government to civilian rule in 1979, but was overcome by a group of junior military officers led by Jerry Rawlings before it could do so. Rawlings allowed elections to be held in 1979, and the government under Ghana's Third Republic functioned haphazardly for a few years before Rawlings was returned to power in yet another military coup in 1981.

Rawlings and his Provisional National Defense Council party saw Ghana through some of its hardest economic times, marked by food shortages, steep inflation, and the accrual of significant debt. Under both internal and external pressure, Rawlings converted his military government to the National Democratic Congress and held democratic elections in 1992. He went on to win both the 1992 and 1996 elections. But in 2000, Ghana's strengthened democratic politics, free media, and increasingly educated populace elected a new political figure, John Agyekum Kufour from the New Patriotic Party. The most recent elections, in 2008, resulted in a peaceful return to power of the National Democratic Congress under John Atta-Mills.

Population

Ghana is a growing nation with a rapidly expanding population, making it one of the most populous countries in West Africa. There are roughly 23.8 million Ghanaians, with 37 percent of the population under the age of fifteen, and an average life expectancy of 58.9 years for males and 60.7 years for females. Ghana is home to an eclectic mix of ethnic groups differentiated by ancestry, language, and religion. The Akan — comprising such notable subgroups as the Fante and Asante — make up almost half of the population (45 percent), thereby influencing many of the country's political, social, and cultural practices. The Mole-Dagbani from the north, the Ewe from the Volta region, and the Ga-Dangme from the southern coast comprise 15 percent, 12 percent, and 7 percent of the population, respectively. Numerous smaller ethnic groups are spread throughout the nation, as are non-African immigrants such as Syrians, Lebanese, and Asians. The capital city of Accra supports a thriving diaspora of Ghanaians returning from all over the world. The official language of the country remains English; the major dialect of the predominant Akan group is Twi. Numerous other dialects and languages are spoken throughout the country, with Ewe, Fante, and Ga among the most popular. With its varied ethnic groups and plethora of languages, Ghana is also home to diverse faiths. Christians comprise 69 percent of the population, with Pentecostal/Charismatic groups making up 24 percent, Protestants nearly 19 percent, Catholics 15 percent, and 11 percent other denominations. There are notable numbers of Muslims (16 percent), located particularly in the north, and another 8.5 percent of the population holds traditional pagan beliefs.

Economy and Income

Over the past two decades in particular, stability and growth have steadily taken hold in Ghana.

The country's per capita gross domestic product (GDP; see the glossary) is U.S. $1,500 (2008 estimate).[1] GDP growth has averaged 4 percent since the mid-1980s, topped 5 percent in 2004 for the first time in a decade, and reached 6.3 percent in 2007. Agriculture is a key economic component, representing 37 percent of the economy and about 56 percent of employment. Cocoa is particularly prominent, accounting for one-third of all exports; Ghana is the world's second largest producer of cocoa.[2] Other cash crops include timber, coconuts, palm products, coffee, and shea butternuts — used to produce shea butter, a vegetable fat.

Ghana's industrial base, which contributes 25 percent of GDP and represents 15 percent of the labor force, is relatively advanced compared to other countries in the region. Mining (mainly of gold and diamonds), hydroelectricity, oil refining, flour milling, and the manufacture of textiles, apparel, beverages, and tobacco are among the leading industries. The services sector accounts for 38 percent of GDP and employs 29 percent of the labor force. Tourism is one of the fastest growing sectors of the economy. In fact, after cocoa, gold, and remittances from abroad, tourism is the country's fourth largest foreign exchange earner.[3] The growth of tourism in Ghana is due in part to the country's political stability and to social, economic, and technological changes that have taken place over time. Tourists are drawn to important events such as the Pan African Festivals, Emancipation Day Celebration, and the National Festival of Arts and Culture. The discovery of major offshore oil reserves, announced in 2007, raised the hopes of a major economic boost in the years to come.[4]

The extent of poverty in Ghana has steadily decreased from 58 percent of the population living in poverty in 2002, to 28.5 percent in 2008. That is, an estimated 28.5 percent of the population lives on less than US$1.00 per day.[5] The government has made significant headway in the fight against poverty and is on track to meet the UN Millennium Development Goal of halving extreme poverty by 2015. However, an expanding urban population, coupled with growing unemployment particularly in cities, continues to pose a challenge in the effort to eliminate poverty. The national unemployment rate is approximately 11 percent.[6] Child labor ranges from 12 percent to 33 percent among five- to seventeen-year-olds, depending on the region.

In the 2003 Core Welfare Indicator Questionnaire survey, conducted by the Ghana Statistical Service, 13 percent of households reported problems meeting basic food needs. Only 11 percent of the population reported using a cooking fuel other than firewood or charcoal. About 42 percent had access to pipe-borne or tanker water, and 33 percent to well or borehole water. While 44 percent of households reported access to electricity, this access was primarily in urban rather than in rural settings (81 percent compared to 25 percent).[7] According to the World Health Organization (WHO; see the glossary), about 15 percent of the population has sustainable access to improved sanitation consisting of sewers, a septic system, or a pit latrine.[8]

Education and Literacy

In Ghana, primary and junior secondary school education is tuition-free and mandatory. The country's commitment to universal access to basic education has been long-standing, dating back to post-independence days when it was against the law to keep a child from attending primary school. Ghana renewed its commitment to education in 1995, when Article 38 was written into the country's constitution.[9] This law requires the government to provide access to free, compulsory, universal, basic education and, depending on resource availability, to senior secondary, technical, and tertiary education and life-long learning. Since 1986, pre-tertiary education in Ghana has included six years of primary education, followed by three years of junior secondary education, and three years at the senior secondary level. Beginning September 2007, educational reform introduced two years of kindergarten education beginning at age four. In addition, senior secondary education was increased from three to four years. The majority of students who pursue that level of education do so at one of the 600 or so public secondary schools. Private secondary schools play a very minor role in Ghana. Successful completion of senior secondary education and an entrance examination make a student eligible to enter one of Ghana's five public universities or one of a handful of training colleges or polytechnic schools.

While Ghana's pre-tertiary education policy is one of the most aggressive in West Africa, significant challenges remain. Access to each successive level of education remains severely limited by lack of facilities, leading to a high level of competition. Although 70 percent of six to eleven-year-olds are enrolled in primary school, secondary school enrollment decreases to about 40 percent of twelve- to seventeen-year-olds. The vast majority (99.1 percent) of junior secondary graduates gain admission to secondary schools; however, only 34 percent of senior secondary graduates are able to gain admission to university and polytechnics. Another 20 percent or so are able to continue on to diploma-level post-secondary schools. Overall, average school life expectancy, or the number of years of schooling is ten years for males and nine years for females.[10]

Although literacy rates in Ghana continue to improve, gender and regional disparities remain. Approximately 58 percent of Ghanaians age fifteen or older can read and write (two-thirds of males and just under half of females).[11] The majority (70 percent) of individuals in urban settings are literate, compared to 40 percent of those in rural settings. Secondary school enrollment is much higher in urban compared to rural areas (51 percent versus 29 percent).[12]

Nearly one-third of Ghanaians have access to the Internet.[13] Radio continues to be Ghana's most popular medium for public education, news, and exchange of ideas, although it is being challenged by the increasing access to televisions.

The Health Care System in Ghana

According to the World Health Organization's 2000 analysis of the world's health systems, Ghana ranks 135th out of 191 member states. (To help put this figure in context, the U.S. healthcare system was ranked 37th by the same report.)[14] Viewed within a regional context, Ghana ranks ninth among countries in sub-Saharan Africa (which excludes North Africa). It is important to point out that this first-ever analysis of the world's health systems used some novel measurements, with the ultimate ranking based on five indicators: overall level of population health; health inequalities, or disparities, within the population; overall level of health system responsiveness; distribution of responsiveness within the population; and distribution of the health system's financial burden within the population.

After independence, Ghana's healthcare system was modeled roughly on Britain's nationalized health care system. Under that model, the government bore most of the cost of healthcare, with the patient paying only a nominal fee at point-of-care. Administratively, the system is organized into the Ghana Health Services, established in 1996, which provides administrative oversight for health services delivery at the national, regional, district, and community level; and the Ghana Ministry of Health, which focuses on health policy and program development. In addition to these governmental agencies, Ghana has four major teaching hospitals: the University of Ghana's affiliated Korle Bu Teaching Hospital, the University of Science and Technology's Komfo Anokye Hospital, the University of Cape Coast's University Hospital, and Tamale Hospital. These teaching hospitals receive referrals from local health posts and from district and regional hospitals. Health services delivery occurs in primary care health posts throughout the country. Ghanaians can also access healthcare at a number of private and mission hospitals. The latter provide a combination of fee-for-service and charity care, while private hospitals operate almost exclusively on a fee-for-service basis. Private health insurance is rare and plays an insignificant role in healthcare financing or private healthcare expenditure.

Over the years, some shifts in healthcare funding have occurred. As national priorities shifted with successive government administrations, Ghana gradually moved away from its post-independence, heavily government-subsidized model of healthcare financing. By the mid-1980s, a different model of financing—a "cash and carry" approach—began to emerge and operated alongside the nationalized model. With the cost of healthcare, medical supplies, and pharmaceuticals rising, the cost of healthcare was steadily shifted away from the government and onto patients and families. As a result, many preventable deaths occurred because the poor delayed seeking care for serious medical conditions. This shift in cost bearing has also been blamed for significant widening of healthcare disparities in the country. For instance, differential access to maternal care services increased between the rich and the poor, the educated and the uneducated; a growing percentage of deliveries occurred in the absence of a skilled birth attendant, and often after little or no prenatal care. Infant mortality and maternal mortality both remained unacceptably high.

Ghana has made some important strides since the 2000 WHO report on health systems. In 2003, Ghana implemented a national HIV/AIDS treatment program, thanks in large part to funding from the Global Fund to Fight AIDS, Tuberculosis and Malaria (see the glossary). Ghana introduced a National Health Insurance Scheme in 2006; it is now estimated that 55 percent of the population has been enrolled. Guided by the Millennium Development Goals, the country has introduced a number of initiatives aimed at reducing infant mortality and improving maternal health. For instance, beginning in 2008, the government extended free medical care to all pregnant women.

Despite these gains, Ghana still faces significant challenges in its healthcare sector. Shortage and distribution of healthcare workers are two of the most challenging issues. With a total of 3,240 physicians, Ghana has an average physician density of 20 per 100,000 population[15]—an inadequate number of physicians to address the healthcare needs of the country. Therefore, a major proportion of the population's healthcare needs are addressed by non-physician health professionals: nurses, pharmacists, public health workers, dispensers or pharmacy assistants, as well as traditional, or non-allopathic, practitioners. However, the distribution of healthcare workers remains uneven, with rural areas relatively underserved compared to urban centers. Expanding pockets of urban poverty have created barriers to accessing health services for some urban populations, comparable to those of many rural areas.

The shortage of healthcare workers has been further exacerbated by a significant brain drain of physicians and nurses from the country. It has been estimated that nearly one-third of the healthcare professionals trained in Ghana (with the assistance of government educational subsidies) currently practice outside the country. An estimated 3,157 health professionals left Ghana between 1993 and 2002, including over 30 percent of all the health professionals trained in the country during this time, with doctors being more likely to leave than nurses.[16] Countries in Europe, Great Britain, and the United States are among the most popular destinations for these Ghanaian emigrants. Graduates of foreign medical schools constitute 33 percent of the total physician workforce in the United Kingdom and 27 percent in the United States. The bulk of these graduates come from lower-income countries; Ghana is among the top contributing countries of medical graduates making up the U.K. and U.S. physician workforce.[17] WHO has identified Ghana on its list of countries with a critical shortage of healthcare workers.[18] Addressing the pressing issue of workforce capacity will continue to be a challenge in the absence of a comprehensive and multilateral solution to the problem of the brain drain.

The shortage of physicians and other health professionals has implications both for access to care and for the type of services available in Ghana. Currently, there is heavy emphasis on acute medical care, and less attention to preventive care or chronic care management. A typical patient in Ghana seeks medical care only when he or she has symptoms, and often after an attempt either to self-treat or to seek alternative, non-allopathic interventions. As a result, patients often present for initial care with advanced symptoms. Physicians are also focused on the care of acute illnesses as a matter of practicality, given the sheer volume of patients and level of acuity of illness that characterize their typical patient load. There have been ongoing efforts to increase health education and early detection of common disorders such as hypertension, diabetes, hepatitis B, malaria, and HIV. Free screening clinics are increasingly common, particularly in urban areas. However, the healthcare system's limited capacity for follow-up care hampers efforts to significantly expand early detection efforts. These challenges are magnified in rural and remote areas where the shortage of healthcare providers is typically worse than in urban centers.

Another barrier to care has been the out-of-pocket expenses borne by the patient; these can include a significant proportion of the cost of ancillary care and diagnostic testing. The newly developed National Health Insurance Scheme is an attempt to cover the cost not only of direct medical care but also of ancillary services. For the nearly half of the population that is not enrolled in the scheme, seeking medical care can be an expensive proposition and one that often necessitates approaching family members, friends, or loan sharks for financial assistance. Many poor patients who do not have access to financial help from family members will choose to ride out their serious illness, often with tragic consequences.

Cultural Considerations in Healthcare Utilization

As in any culture, several other factors play an important role in an individual Ghanaian's utilization of healthcare, over and above the availability and accessibility of healthcare services. Level of education, socioeconomic status, cultural and religious beliefs, and social support systems affect an individual's perception of health and disease in general, the perceived need for healthcare, and the ability to seek out such care.[19]

When walking through the streets of cities such as Accra and Kumasi, you are likely to see various faith-related messages posted on shop fronts, vegetable stands, backs of taxis, and even some waiting areas. Given the overriding influence of religion on the social fabric of Ghana, it is not surprising that religion would also have an impact on health beliefs, practices, and utilization of care.[20] Congregations, as well as tribal leaders, can play a significant role in community health education, in delivering programs, and in developing social support systems for persons with diseases such as HIV.[21] In some circumstances societal beliefs may contribute to stigma. For instance, infection with HIV/AIDS is widely viewed in Ghana as being a result of immoral behavior.[22]

Approximately 80 percent of the population in Africa uses traditional medicine for health care.[23] Traditional medical practices are often used instead of or in combination with Western medicine, and can be the most affordable and accessible form of healthcare, especially for the poor and those in rural areas. In Africa, the ratio of traditional healers to population is 250 per 100,000, while the ratio of medical doctors to population is 20 per 100,000.[24] Many traditional healers are priests and priestesses of deities who use divination and ritual techniques to treat diseases. Diseases are thought to be either organic or spiritually based.[25] As an example, many individuals do not believe in the mosquito theory of transmission of lymphatic filariasis (a disease marked by the presence of adult worms in the lymphatics), but rather attribute the disease to other physical, spiritual, or hereditary causes.[26] Some Ghanaians believe in *juju* (black magic) that can harm or help a person, including in the area of health. Other types of traditional healers and practitioners include sacred healers (who are faith healers whose treatment techniques include prayers, fasting, incantations, and herbal medicines), secular healers (also known as traditional pharmacists), and plant drug peddlers.

The health status of women and their empowerment in society can have a significant impact on the health of families and society at large. Food-related superstitions and other food restrictions on women of childbearing age in general, and pregnant and lactating women in particular, along with the traditional practice of serving the best part of the meal to the male members of the household can worsen the health of women in a society.[27] Women with limited education and few vocational skills may take on boyfriends to help support them as a means of economic security.[28] However, even in these relationships, condom use may be avoided for reasons that can include the high value placed on fertility, the association of condoms with prostitution, and the limited ability of women to influence decision-making in this area. Overall, contraceptive use is relatively low, probably due to negative socio-cultural perceptions (for instance, married women who use contraceptives may be suspected of having an extramarital sexual relationship).[29] In rural Ghana, home birth has been found to elevate a woman's status in her community, while having a skilled attendant at the delivery lowers it.[30]

As in many societies, financial accessibility can impact the use of healthcare. While healthcare in Ghana has primarily been fee-for-service, there is now the potential for increased utilization of health-care services with enrollment in Ghana's relatively new National Health Insurance Scheme. One study of over 2,000 Ghanaian children showed that a prepayment scheme allowing free primary care does increase use of children's health services compared to the normal fee-for-service practices.[31] Greater utilization may also be contingent upon increasing understanding of the concept of health insurance, a shift in focus to prevention rather than treatment, and a growing empowerment of Ghanaians in their healthcare and in traditionally paternalistic doctor-patient relationships.

Leading Health and Environmental Issues in Ghana

The leading causes of death in Ghana are typical of sub-Saharan Africa: HIV/AIDS, malaria, lower respiratory infections, perinatal conditions, cerebrovascular diseases, ischemic heart disease, and diarrheal diseases.[32] In addition, 3 percent of all deaths in Ghana are due to motor vehicle accidents. Tobacco use, with a prevalence rate of 11.7 percent, is a leading risk factor for the majority of non-communicable causes of death in adulthood.

HIV/AIDS

Compared to the region, Ghana's HIV prevalence rate of 1.7 percent is relatively low. HIV/AIDS accounts for 131 deaths per 100,000 population.[33] Because of its disproportionate burden on adults between the ages of fifteen and forty-nine, HIV/AIDS has both a direct human toll and huge implications for economic development. Over the past decade, Ghana has made significant strides in its efforts to stem the tide of HIV/AIDS. A relatively aggressive campaign to educate the public about the risks for exposure to HIV/AIDS and the benefits of early detection has begun to pay off. These prevention and education efforts received a further boost in 2003, when Ghana launched its national treatment program with support from the Global Fund to Fight AIDS, Tuberculosis and Malaria (see the glossary). In 2004, it was estimated that 79,000 people living with HIV/AIDS in Ghana needed antiretroviral therapy (ART; see the glossary), but only 3 percent of them were actually receiving it.[34] This increased to 15 percent by 2007, but still represents a small proportion of those who are in need of ART. The pace of progress has been similarly slow in the area of prevention of mother-to-child transmission (PMTCT; see the glossary). Although significant strides have been made since 2004, when only 1 percent of pregnant women living with HIV received antiretrovirals, the majority (roughly 80 percent) of women needing therapy still do not receive it.

Stigma remains a significant barrier to HIV testing and treatment. However, thanks to initiatives by governmental agencies as well as nongovernmental and community-based organizations, stigma reduction interventions have seen signs of success. More Ghanaians are open to seeking voluntary counseling and testing than ever before, but much more work needs to be done in this area. Fear of stigmatization continues to keep too many Ghanaians from seeking early testing and treatment.

Malaria

Malaria (see the glossary) is a leading health problem in Ghana, with an estimated 7.2 million cases each year.[35] Malaria accounts for one in every four deaths in children under five, making it the leading cause of death in children. Most cases are caused by *Plasmodium falciparum*, although diagnostic confirmation occurs in only 10 percent to 15 percent of cases. The bulk of suspected malaria in children and adults is treated presumptively, without diagnostic confirmation, and at home. Sixty-three percent of all febrile children receive treatment for malaria, although only 4 percent receive first-line treatment of artemisinin-based combination therapy. For many people with suspected malaria, the first line of care is through a licensed chemical seller or drug dispenser. Because of this reality, efforts have been made to train these dispensers to recognize the signs and symptoms of malaria and to know when to refer someone to the hospital.

WHO recommendations for the prevention of malaria include the use of insecticide-treated bed nets. Bed nets are distributed free to families with children under five and to pregnant women as part of an international effort to halve the burden of malaria by the year 2015. Still, recent surveys suggest that only 19 percent of households own at least one insecticide-treated bed net.[36] Other effective interventions for reducing the impact of malaria include use of a long-lasting insecticidal bed net (as opposed to nets that need to be retreated every six to twelve months), indoor residual spraying with insecticides, and use of first-line therapy with artemisinin-based combination treatment for suspected cases of malaria.

Tuberculosis

Approximately 48,000 new cases of tuberculosis (TB; see the glossary) are diagnosed each year in Ghana, an incidence rate of 203 cases per 100,000 population; the overall prevalence rate is 379 cases per 100,000 population.[37] Significant improvement through surveillance and treatment of tuberculosis over a number of years has since been undermined by the HIV epidemic. Death from TB among persons who are HIV-negative has steadily declined since 1990.[38] In contrast, from 1990 through the mid-1990s, the TB-related death rate among people who were HIV-positive rose from 1.0 to 7.0 per 100,000 population. The death rate remained at the new high until 2005, when it began to decline, most likely due to the increased availability of HIV/AIDS treatment. Directly observed therapy (part of the DOTS strategy; see the glossary) is used throughout the country to treat TB patients, and the coverage is estimated to be 100 percent.

Traffic-Related Accidents

Traffic accidents are an important contributing factor to premature death, and a growing public health problem in Ghana. In fact, road safety and traffic-related injuries are serious public health issues in many African and low-income countries around the globe. Ghana is no exception. Motor vehicle–associated fatality rates in Ghana are thirty to forty times greater than those in industrialized countries.[39] Excessive speeding on highways and in highly congested areas has been blamed for a large proportion of traffic accidents. The use of speed bumps has significantly reduced fatalities.[40] For example, following the construction of rumble strips on the main Accra-Kumasi highway, traffic accidents fell by about 35 percent.

Road safety is further hampered by lack of an adequate public transportation system, a problem that plagues many low-income countries. Informal modes of transportation—privately owned cars, minibuses, converted pick-up trucks and buses—have emerged to fill the gap created by inadequate public transportation. The low fares charged by these vehicles, referred to as *tro tros* in Ghana, make them affordable, especially to the poor. However, there is a lack of uniformity in their safety. Vehicles are typically packed far beyond their capacity with passengers and goods, and passengers often precariously perch on the rooftops or cling to the sides of vehicles. Drivers often work long hours, and their fatigue can cause hazardous driving. Another source of traffic-related fatalities is crashes between vehicles and pedestrians. Pedestrian accident–related injuries involving children, in particular, is a major and growing problem as the number of vehicles on the road increase.

The lack of adequate infrastructure for emergency and trauma care in Ghana and other low-income countries is a major contributing problem to traffic fatalities. This lack of infrastructure significantly reduces the chances of surviving a serious motor vehicle accident. In Ghana, as in many low-income countries, rescue by ambulance is rare. Most accident victims who make it to the hospital do so in a commercial or private vehicle, with the only form of pre-hospital care being assistance from lay bystanders. Therefore, pre-hospital mortality is very high. Even if an accident victim makes it to the hospital, the chance of survival is further hampered by the lack of sufficient numbers of trained surgeons. A study based at a main hospital in Kumasi found an average delay of twelve hours before initiation of emergency surgery. The lack of essential, low-cost, and reusable equipment is a further barrier to effective emergency care. A survey of eleven rural hospitals in Ghana found that none stocked chest tubes (used to re-expand collapsed lungs), and only four had emergency airway equipment. The study determined that this lack of key equipment was due to poor planning rather than to cost considerations.[41]

Agencies and Organizations Working in Ghana

Ghana is home to hundreds of local and international NGOs engaged in health-related work. Most international aid and development agencies have country and regional offices located in Accra, the capital. Agencies such as the U.S. Agency for International Development (USAID; see the glossary), the United Kingdom's Department for International Development (DFID), and various UN agencies (including the World Food Program; UNICEF and UNAIDS [see the glossary for both]; and the Population Council) all have programs targeting aspects of public health in Ghana. It is generally useful to investigate which, if any, organizations are working in your destination area prior to traveling to Ghana. While an exhaustive list of agencies and organizations doing work in Ghana is beyond the scope of this chapter, mentioning a few representative organizations will give you an idea of different approaches to global health work in Ghana. In addition, we share some of the work with which we have been most closely involved — the Foundation for African Relief.

Family Health International is one of the most active organizations operating in Ghana in the area of public health education and research. The organization has programs addressing the needs of people living with HIV/AIDS, prevention of mother-to-child transmission of HIV, TB, malaria, and other infectious and chronic diseases in Ghana.

Noguchi Memorial Institute for Medical Research, a biomedical research institution in Ghana, is among the leading medical institutions in Africa. Founded in 1979, it is located on the campus of the University of Ghana (Legon campus). The facilities were built by the government of Japan as a gift to Ghana in honor of Hideyo Noguchi, a medical scientist who died in Ghana while researching yellow fever. The institute's areas of research include communicable diseases and nutrition. It receives funding from a number of international agencies as well as the Ghana government.

Conclusion

Ghana has long been an attractive destination for global health and development workers. This is in part because of its rich history, geopolitical stability, and historical ties to the developed world. Ghana has made important strides over the last decade and is well poised to continue to play a leading role in sub-Saharan Africa. Despite the presence of challenges in the health and educational sectors, there is ample opportunity for the global health worker choosing to work in Ghana to make a difference.

Careful planning and preparation are key first steps to embarking on work in Ghana. Choosing a project that is realistic for your given time frame — taking into account that unanticipated challenges may arise — is especially critical. Be proactive before you arrive in Ghana to reach out to local collaborators for help in planning your project, and discuss whether you will need an interpreter to work effectively. Once you arrive in the country you will find most Ghanaians very hospitable and eager to help you. Many will be curious and call out to you on the

THE FOUNDATION FOR AFRICAN RELIEF
A Collaborative Approach to Improving Access to Health Care

The NGO Foundation for African Relief (FAR) was co-founded in 2000 by one of the authors of this chapter, Joyce Sackey, along with Deborah Morris-Harris and Kwaku Acheampong, with a goal of fostering collaboration between health professionals in the United States and their Ghanaian counterparts to address disparities in access to health care in Ghana.

The AIDS Collaborative Project, FAR's first initiative, was launched in 2001. This project empowers health care professionals in Ghana caring for people living with HIV/AIDS by providing the medical resources, education, and training they need to effectively care for their patients. Through a collaborative effort with Beth Israel Deaconess Medical Center (BIDMC), a Harvard Medical School–affiliated hospital in Boston, FAR offers faculty development opportunities for Ghanaian physicians who participate as visiting scholars in a program to develop HIV/AIDS care and management skills. During the ten- to twelve-week-long program, visiting scholars spend time with physicians in Boston-based clinical settings learning initial evaluation of patients newly diagnosed with HIV, how to initiate antiretroviral therapy, critical skills in monitoring patients on therapy, how to enhance adherence to therapy, and the treatment and prevention of opportunistic infections. Visiting scholars also select an aspect of HIV care for in-depth study under the mentorship of an expert and give an oral presentation on their independent study at a hospital conference, including specific plans to apply their newly acquired knowledge to the care of patients upon their return to Ghana. To facilitate post-program learning and collaboration, each scholar receives a laptop upon program completion and is encouraged to keep in touch with preceptors and mentors in Boston after returning to Ghana. Post-program opportunities and collaborative efforts often lead to publications and presentations at international conferences.

The first two physicians to participate in the visiting scholars program, Peter Preko and George Frimpong, returned to Ghana and co-founded AIDS ALLY, a Ghana-based nonprofit organization that creates a comprehensive model of care for people living with HIV/AIDS. In a collaborative effort with FAR, AIDS ALLY opened the first clinic in Kumasi to provide comprehensive HIV/AIDS care and support. Within months of opening its doors, the clinic had hundreds of patients on ART and was receiving referrals from area health centers. It was clear that the needs of the community far exceeded the capacity of the clinic. AIDS ALLY and FAR have collaborated to co-sponsor train-the-trainer workshops on HIV/AIDS management for health provider groups in Kumasi and Accra, in an effort to increase local expertise in HIV/AIDS care. Over two hundred physicians, pharmacists, nurses, and nurse midwives from health districts throughout Ghana participated in these workshops, led by local Ghanaian physician leaders and Harvard Medical School faculty. These efforts helped to create a critical mass of health professionals within Ghana with expertise in HIV/AIDS treatment well before Ghana introduced a national treatment program in 2003. With the establishment of the Global Fund to Fight AIDS, Tuberculosis and Malaria, Ghana was finally in a position to offer comprehensive care to people living with HIV/AIDS. The original AIDS ALLY comprehensive HIV/AIDS clinic in Kumasi became the model for the national treatment program.

In the summer of 2008, FAR initiated a mobile healthcare clinic in a rural area of Ghana as well as the poorer neighborhoods in Accra. Assembling a team of five Ghanaian physicians, seven physicians from Harvard, three Ghanaian nurses and two pharmacists, the clinic set up in local schools to address the acute healthcare needs of the community, as well as to offer screening for HIV and hepatitis infection. By partnering with a local church and community leaders, the mobile clinic outreach served over 2,000 patients in a week. Because Ghanaian physicians were present on-site, each patient needing follow-up care was referred to a specific clinic that would provide such care, an especially critical component for those who tested positive for HIV. In addition to connecting patients to the healthcare system, individuals could enroll on-site for the National Health Insurance Scheme. FAR had raised money in advance to assist with payment of premiums, assuring patients both financial and practical access to the health system.

street, "*Obronee*," meaning foreigner. When asked, be wise and cautious about giving out your contact information. Acquiring a local cell phone is a good idea for communication and safety if traveling independently.

Great respect and deference is given to individuals of higher rank in Ghanaian society, both within and outside of the tribal system. Therefore, try to build relationships and gain the trust of local leaders before embarking upon your project. Be mindful of the implicit rank given to you as well. Females, younger individuals, and trainees taking on leadership roles may need to work especially carefully on building relationships in order to be respected in working collaborations. Face-to-face meetings are always best for effective communication. Be aware that meetings may not start at their scheduled times; many formalities may need to be exchanged, and there will be continued emphasis on relationship building. People may be more likely to provide you with honest input and feedback one-on-one than in groups. Over time, if you would like to discuss areas for improvement, try to do so in a positive way that sparks further communication on how to address these areas jointly. Otherwise, local collaborators might assume they should immediately try to fix on their own the problems that you raise.

Workers who pay close attention to a community-centered, collaborative approach and adopt a flexible, open-minded attitude are likely to find success in their work and to have a fulfilling and enjoyable time in this relatively small, yet unforgettable country.

Millennium Development Goal indicators are italicized.

TABLE 4.1 : **POPULATION AND HUMAN DEVELOPMENT**

POPULATION	
Total	23.8 million
Population growth rate	1.88%
Net migration rate/1,000 population	−0.53
Urban	50%
Rural	50%
AGE STRUCTURE	
0–14 years	37.3%
15–64 years	59.1%
65+ years	3.6%
Median age (years)	20.7
MAJOR ETHNIC GROUPS	
Akan	45%
Mole-Dagbon	15%
Ewe	12%
Ga-Dangme	7%
Other	28%
RELIGIONS	
Christian	69%
Muslim	16%
Indigenous/traditional	8.5%
Other	0.7%
None	6.6%
HUMAN DEVELOPMENT	
Human Development Index	0.533
Human Development rank[a]	142nd
Freedom House Index	Free
Political Rights score[b]	1
Civil Liberties score[b]	2
Human Poverty Index	32.3%
Human Poverty rank[c]	65th

Notes: [a]out of 179 countries; [b]1 = most free, 7 = least free; [c]out of 135 developing countries

TABLE 4.2 : **GOVERNMENT AND ECONOMY**

GOVERNMENT

Independence	6 Mar. 1957 from Britain
Type of government	Constitutional democracy
Voting rights	Age 18, universal

CAPITAL — Accra

CURRENCY — Ghana cedi (GHC)

ECONOMY

Gross Domestic Product (GDP) (in PPP US $)	$34.04 billion
Annual GDP growth	6.3%
GDP Per Capita (in US $)	$1,500
Gini Index	39.4
Population living below PPP $1/day	*28.5%*
Public debt as % of GDP	62.3
Official Development Assistance (ODA) per capita (in US $)	NA
Foreign direct investment as % of GDP	1.0

LABOR FORCE

In agriculture	56%
In industry	15%
In services	29%
Unemployment rate	11%

TABLE 4.3 : **GEOGRAPHY AND ENVIRONMENT**

LAND COMPOSITION

Land area	239,460 sq. km. (92,456 sq. mi.)
Size comparison	Slightly smaller than Oregon
Terrain	Low plains; plateau in south-central area; 539-km (335-mi.) coastline along Gulf of Guinea
Ecological hazards	Droughts; dry, dusty winds January–March

LAND USE AND RESOURCES

Permanent crop land	9.22%
Arable land	17.54%
Agricultural products	Cocoa, rice, cassava, peanuts, corn, bananas
Natural resources	Gold, timber, industrial diamonds, bauxite, manganese, fish, rubber, hydropower, petroleum, silver, salt, limestone

ENVIRONMENTAL ISSUES Soil erosion, drought in north, deforestation, overgrazing, poaching, water pollution, inadequate supply of potable water

INFRASTRUCTURE

Population without access to improved water source	80%
Population using improved sanitation	15%
Roadways unpaved	84%

TABLE 4.4 : **HEALTH**

LIFE, BIRTH, DEATH

Life expectancy at birth (male/female)	58.9/60.7
Birth rate/1,000 population	28.58
Death rate/1,000 population	9.24
Infant mortality rate/1,000 live births	*51.09*

PERSONNEL AND INFRASTRUCTURE

Physicians/100,000 population	20
Hospital beds/10,000 population	9

HEALTH ECONOMICS

Total expenditure on health per capita (PPP US $)	$95
Public expenditure on health as % of GDP	2.8

DISEASES

Most common vector-borne diseases	Malaria, yellow fever
Most common food- and water-borne diseases	Bacterial/protozoal diarrhea, hepatitis A, typhoid fever, schistosomiasis
TB incidence/100,000 population	*203*
TB prevalence/100,000 population	*379*
New TB cases HIV-positive	7%
New TB cases multidrug-resistant (MDR)	1.9%
1-year-olds fully immunized against TB	99%
Estimated malaria cases annually	7.3 million
Malaria death rate/100,000 population	NA
HIV prevalence rate in adults	*1.7%*
AIDS deaths in adults annually	*21,000*
People living with HIV	260,000
AIDS orphans	170,000

MATERNAL HEALTH

Fertility rate (children born per woman)	3.68
Contraceptive prevalence rate (married women 15–49)	*25%*
Maternal mortality rate/100,000 births	*560*
Lifetime risk of maternal death, 1 in:	*45*
Births attended by skilled birth attendant	*47%*

CHILD HEALTH

Mortality rate of children < 5/1,000 live births	*120*
1-year-olds immunized against measles	*85%*
Children < 5 using insecticide-treated bed nets	*22%*

Children < 5 with fever treated with antimalarial drugs	63%
Newborns protected against tetanus	86%

HUNGER AND MALNUTRITION

Children < 5 underweight for age	22%
Children < 5 under height for age	36%
Population undernourished	11%

TABLE 4.5 : **LANGUAGE, EDUCATION, AND LITERACY**

LANGUAGES

English (offical language)	
Asante (Twi is predominant dialect)	15%
Ewe	13%
Fante	10%
Other (including Boron, Dagomba, Dangme, Dagarte)	63%

LITERACY

Adult literacy rate (population age 15+ who can read and write)	57.9%

EXPENDITURE

Public expenditure on education as % of GDP	5.4

EDUCATION

Primary mandatory	Yes
Secondary mandatory	No
Net enrollment in primary education[d]	71.9%
School life expectancy, in years (male/female)[e]	10/9

[d]Net enrollment rate in primary education is measured as the number of children of official primary school age who are enrolled in primary education as a percentage of children in the official primary school age population.

[e]School life expectancy is the total number of years of school (from primary through tertiary education) that a child can expect to receive.

Principal Sources for Data in Appendix Tables 4.1–4.5

Central Intelligence Agency, *The World Factbook* (https://www.cia.gov/library/publications/the-world-factbook/).

UN Millennium Development Goals Indicators Database (www.mdgs.un.org).

UNDP Human Development Report, 2007/2008 (www.hdrstats.undp.org).

WHO. Global Tuberculosis Control. WHO Report 2008.

1. Central Intelligence Agency, The World Factbook. Ghana. (https://www.cia.gov/library/publications/the-world-factbook/geos/gh.html).

2. BBC News. Country Profile: Ghana. http://news.bbc.co.uk/2/hi/africa/country_profiles/1023355.stm).

3. Ghana Statistical Service (http://www.statsghana.gov.gh/TourismMarket.html).

4. BBC News. Country Profile: Ghana.

5. World Food Programme. Ghana. 2010. (http://www.wfp.org/node/3467).

6. Central Intelligence Agency, The World Factbook, Ghana.

7. Ghana Statistical Service, "2003 Core Welfare Indicators Questionnaire (CWIQ) Survey, Ghana: National Summary" (http://www.statsghana.gov.gh/docfiles/cwiq%20%20nat.pdf). This survey provides information on several factors likely to have a significant impact on public health. This nationwide sample survey, the second of its kind in Ghana (the first was in 1997) was designed to provide indicators for monitoring poverty and living standards in the country, at national, regional and district levels. It uses a district-based probability sample that covered a total of 49,003 households nationwide, with 405 households drawn from each district, except for the metropolitan areas where samples were larger.

8. WHO/UNICEF, "Joint Monitoring Programme for Water Supply and Sanitation: Coverage Estimates; Improved Sanitation—Ghana" (July 2008; http://www.childinfo.org/files/GHA_san.pdf).

9. Central Intelligence Agency, The World Factbook. Ghana.

10. Ibid.

11. Ibid.

12. BBC News. Country Profile: Ghana.

13. Ibid.

14. World Health Organization, "The World Health Report 2000—Health Systems: Improving Performance" (http://www.who.int/whr/2000/en/).

15. Research Africa, Country Information, Ghana, 2010 (http://researchafrica.rti.org/index.cfm?fuseaction=home.country_view&country_id=16#ntl-hlth-policy).

16. World Health Organization, "The World Health Report 2006—Working Together for Health" (http://www.who.int/whr/2006/en/index.html).

17. Fitzhugh Mullan, "The Metrics of the Physician Brain Drain," *New England Journal of Medicine* 353 (2005): 1810-18.

18. World Health Organization, "The World Health Report 2006."

19. M. Tabi, M. Powell, and D. Hodnicki, "Use of Traditional Healers and Modern Medicine in Ghana," *International Nursing Review* 53, no. 1 (2006): 52-58.

20. S. O. Gyimah, K. T. Baffour, and I. Addai, "Challenges to the Reproductive-health Needs of African Women: On Religion and Maternal Health Utilization in Ghana," *Social Science & Medicine* 62 (2006): 2930–44; I. N. Luginaah, E. K. Yiridoe, M. M. Taabazuing, "From Mandatory to Voluntary Testing: Balancing Human Rights, Religious and Cultural Values, and HIV/AIDS Prevention in Ghana," *Social Science & Medicine* 61 (2005): 1689–1700; I. Addai, "Determinants of Use of Maternal-Child Health Services in Rural Ghana," *Journal of Biosocial Sciences* 32 (2000): 1–15.

21. E. S. Bazant, M. Boulay, "Factors Associated with Religious Congregation Members' Support to People Living with HIV/AIDS in Kumasi, Ghana," *AIDS and Behavior* 1 (2007): 936–45.

22. C. I. Ulasi, et al., "HIV/AIDS-related Stigma in Kumasi, Ghana," *Health & Place* 15 (2009):255–62.

23. Leah Patterson, "2nd Annual International Conference on Traditional Medicine in Ghana, Africa," *Holistic Times* 8, no. 4 (2001): 10–12 (http://www .ccnh.edu/community/newsletter/holtimesv8n4/fp_v8n4.aspx); World Health Organization, Regional Office for Africa, "Traditional Medicine Meeting Ends, Makes Recommendations" (24 November 2004; http://www.afro.who.int/en/ media-centre/notes-for-the-press/413-traditional-medicine-meeting-ends-makes-recommendations-.html).

24. Patterson, "2nd Annual International Conference."

25. Tabi, Powell, and Hodnicki, "Use of Traditional Healers and Modern Medicine in Ghana."

26. C. K. Ahorlu, et al., "Lymphatic Filariasis Related Perceptions and Practices on the Coast of Ghana: Implications for Prevention and Control," *Acta Tropica* 73 (1999): 251–64.

27. SH Mayhew, "Integration of STI Services into FP/MCH Services: Health Service and Social Contexts in Rural Ghana." *Reproductive Health Matters* 8 (2000): 112–24.

28. J. E. Mill and J. K. Anarfi, "HIV Risk Environment for Ghanaian Women: Challenges to Prevention," *Social Science & Medicine* 54 (2002): 325–37.

29. Olivia Kwapong, "The Health Situation of Women in Ghana," *Rural and Remote Health* 8 (2008):963 (http://www.rrh.org.au/articles/subviewnew.asp ?articleID=963).

30. A. N. Bazzano et al., "Social Costs of Skilled Attendance at Birth in Rural Ghana," *International Journal of Gynecology and Obstetrics* 102 (2008): 91–94.

31. E. Ansah et al., "Effect of Removing Direct Payment for Health Care on Utilization and Health Outcomes in Ghanaian Children: A Randomised Control Trial," *PLoS Medicine* (2009; http://www.plosmedicine.org/article/info%3Adoi %2F10.1371%2Fjournal.pmed.100000).

32. BBC News. Country Profile: Ghana.

33. UNAIDS/WHO. Global HIV/AID Online Database. Epidemiological Fact Sheets on HIV/AIDS and Sexually Transmitted Infections. Ghana. (2010; Apps.who.int/GlobalAtlas/predefinedReports/EFS2008/index.asp ?strSelectedCounty=gH).

34. World Health Organization, "The World Health Report 2006—Working Together for Health" (http://www.who.int/whr/2006/en/index.html).

35. World Health Organization, Ghana. Data from the Global Health Observatory (2010. http://apps.who.int/ghodata/?vid=9300).

36. Ibid.

37. World Health Organization, "Tuberculosis (TB) Country Profiles" (http://www.who.int/tb/country/global_tb_database/en/index2.html).

38. BBC News. Country Profile: Ghana.

39. World Health Organization, "World Report on Road Traffic Injury Prevention" (Geneva: WHO, 2004; http://www.who.int/violence_injury_prevention/publications/road_traffic/world_report/en/index.html).

40. Ibid.

41. Ibid.

SUGGESTED READING

Central Intelligence Agency. The World Factbook. Ghana. (https://www.cia .gov/library/publications/the-world-factbook/geos/gh.html).

Gocking, Roger S. *The History of Ghana*. Westport, Conn.: Greenwood, 2005.

Kwame, Boafo-Arthur. *Ghana: One Decade of the Liberal State*. London: Zed, 2007.

Osei, Akwasi. *Ghana: Recurrence and Change in a Post-Independence African State*. New York: Peter Lang, 1999.

World Health Organization. "Country Cooperation Strategy at a Glance: Ghana." Geneva: WHO, 2009 (http://www.who.int/countryfocus/cooperation _strategy/ccsbrief_gha_en.pdf).

5

STEPHANIE WILLMAN BORDAT

SAIDA KOUZZI

THE MAGHREB

ALGERIA, MOROCCO, AND TUNISIA

Diversity, authenticity, modernity, and specificities are four words that visitors to the Maghreb will hear frequently, whether in promotional tourist materials, political discourse, or development initiatives. This is a region with wide diversity across communities, long-held traditions that impact current-day values and beliefs, struggles between tradition and emerging modern realities, and a strong sense of uniqueness. Travelers to the region should keep these concepts in mind as they design and implement projects. These concepts describe concrete realities of life in the Maghreb and reveal a great deal about regional self-identity and relations with outsiders.

This chapter highlights issues faced by women in a social context where religion plays a role in all behaviors, and tradition encounters modern pressures daily. The chapter presents examples from all three countries in order to highlight differences and encourage reflection on the issues we've raised when you look at other countries.

Maghreb in Arabic refers to the "land of the setting sun," or the westernmost part of the Arab world, as contrasted to the Mashreq, the "land of the rising sun" or Middle East. This chapter uses Maghreb in its geographic sense, to refer to the three countries of Algeria, Morocco, and Tunisia. The term "Greater Maghreb" is used to designate the five countries of the Arab Maghreb Union (Algeria, Morocco, and Tunisia, plus

Mauritania and Libya), created in 1989, to enhance political and economic ties between the countries.

The Maghreb Regional Context

Algeria, Morocco and Tunisia are located in northwest Africa, with the Mediterranean to the north and date palm oases and the Sahara in the south. Morocco opens to the west onto the Atlantic Ocean, and is a mere fourteen kilometers (slightly less than nine miles) across the Strait of Gibraltar from Spain. Several mountain ranges cut across the Maghreb, creating geographically, socially, and culturally distinct communities: in Morocco the Rif, Middle Atlas, High Atlas, and Anti-Atlas; in Algeria the Tell Atlas and Saharan Atlas; and in Tunisia the Dorsal extension of the Atlas Mountains. This diverse geography explains many of the region's main economic activities and revenue sources: agriculture in the plains, including grains, olives, grapes and wine, and citrus fruits; fishing; and phosphate mining. Algeria has a significant oil industry,[1] Morocco and Tunisia profit from tourism and traditional handicrafts, and all three economies have a large portion of income from earnings sent home by their citizens who live and work abroad.

Population
Algeria is the largest of the three countries (2,380,000 square kilometers, or 918,923 square miles, with 34.2 million people, over 80 percent of whom live on the 10 percent of the area along the northern coast), compared to Morocco's 446,550 square kilometers, or 172,433 square miles, with 34.8 million people. Tunisia is the smallest in both size and population, with 10.4 million people in 163,600 square kilometers, or 63,166 square miles. Rural exodus and high urbanization in recent decades have resulted in the majority of the region's population living in urban areas. All three countries experienced high population growth after independence in the middle of the twentieth century, have a high proportion of the population that is young, and have significant rates of out-migration, primarily to Europe.

All three constitutions proclaim Arabic as the official language, although 2002 amendments in Algeria provide that Tamazight[2] is also a "national" language. While modern standard Arabic is used for reading, writing, official use, and broadcast speaking, each country has its own distinct dialect of spoken Arabic with unique vocabulary that differs from town to town and across regions. Likewise, there are numerous distinct dialects of Tamazight in different communities across the Maghreb. French is a commonly spoken second language in all three countries among the urban educated elite. In northern Morocco, spoken Arabic is frequently interspersed with Spanish vocabulary.

Both Morocco and Algeria have ethnically mixed Arab and Amazigh populations; estimates of the Amazigh populations in each country range from 30 percent to over 50 percent. Over the past decade Algeria, in particular, has experienced ethnic tensions and sometimes violent confrontations in the Kabylie region (the northern mountainous region along the Mediterranean) between police and Amazigh populations advocating for political, linguistic, and cultural rights. While Amazigh activism is dynamic and tolerated in Morocco, the Tunisian government has long repressed all movements based on anything other than an Arab identity and denies the existence of any Amazigh population in the country.[3]

All three national constitutions proclaim Islam as the official state religion, with over 98 percent of the populations identified as Muslims, in large majority following the Maliki school of Sunni Islam. Several major religious holidays are strictly observed as national holidays in all three countries. During the month of Ramadan, Muslims are required to refrain from eating, drinking, smoking, and sexual relations from sunrise to sunset, and as a result workday hours are reduced and energy levels are at a low during the day. In contrast, following the breaking of the fast at sunset, the evenings and nights are quite lively and exciting.

While there are apparent differences in religious observance between countries and regions, you should avoid categorizing countries as more or less strict or religiously conservative. Rather, you should take care to distinguish between doctrinal religion (of which there are numerous schools of jurisprudence), official religion as promoted by state institutions,[4] popular religion as practiced by people in their daily lives, and political religion as used by political parties and reactionary groups (discussed later in more detail). Also, there are diverse expressions of religious belief on a wide spectrum of public and private practices that can vary across communities, such as the observance of the five pillars of Islam,[5] the weekend days,[6] debates on using loudspeakers in mosques for the call to prayer,[7] and different laws regulating the sale of alcohol.[8]

Politics and Government

All three countries were colonized by the French and obtained their independence in the mid-twentieth century, after substantially different colonial experiences. Tunisia was made a French protectorate in 1881, and Morocco in 1912; both became independent in 1956. In contrast, the French occupation of Algeria started in 1830 and did not end until 1962, after a bloody eight-year war of independence.

All three countries have highly centralized constitutional governments: Morocco a dynastic monarchy that has ruled since the seventeenth century; Algeria and Tunisia are republics. All three are dominated by very strong executive branches and entrenched power in the bureaucracy, weak legislatures, and judiciaries of limited independence. While Morocco and Algeria have multiparty systems, Tunisia is dominated by a single political party (the Rassemblement Constitutionnel Democratique, or Democratic Constitutional Rally), with only 20 percent of the seats in the Chamber of Deputies reserved for representatives from the few authorized opposition parties, frequently referred to by local activists as the "pseudo-opposition." Tunisia has had only two presidents since independence. The current president, Zine El Abidine Ben Ali, in power since 1987, was reelected in 2004 with 99 percent of votes and again in 2009 in another landslide. Constitutional reforms in 2002, eliminating the presidential three-term limit and raising the age limit to seventy-five, seem to ensure him a fourth term that will last through 2014.

In Algeria, the military establishment has traditionally had a strong influence on defense, foreign policy, and internal politics. October 2008 constitutional reforms eliminated term limits for the presidency, and in April 2009 President Abdelaziz Bouteflika was reelected for a third term with 90 percent of votes.

In Morocco, the powerful king is both the head of state (political leader) and the commander of the faithful (religious authority). Mohammed VI, became king in 1999 and has promoted a platform of democratization and progressive reforms. He set up an Equity and Reconciliation Commission (now defunct) to document human rights abuses perpetrated under his late father, Hassan II, who ruled from 1961 to 1999. In the September 2007 national parliamentary elections, the traditional centrist Istiqlal (independence) Party emerged as the single largest party in the parliament, while the "moderate Islamist" Justice and Development Party became the second largest party. A new political party created in 2008, (Parti Authenticité et Modernité, or the Authenticity and Modernity Party) united several political parties and is now the largest party in Parliament, with the Istiqlal second and the Justice and Development Party third.

Algeria and Morocco have long-standing tensions due to conflict over the western Sahara, with Morocco claiming the western Sahara as part of its kingdom and Algeria recognizing an independent Polisario government. In the fall of 2005, a group of Moroccan prisoners of war who had been held for decades in Polisario camps in Tindouf were released. A UN referendum on self-determination of the Polisario region, originally scheduled for 1992, has yet to be held. Thus, a solution to the issue of independence of the region versus autonomy under Morocco is still pending.

Growing Religious Extremism

Over the past two decades, all three countries of the Maghreb have had to confront both growing violence based on religious extremism and allow for political parties based on religion. In January 2007, a network of militant organizations declared itself to be Al-Qaeda Maghreb and its intention to conduct terrorist attacks in the region.

The Tunisian government has been severely criticized for its repression of Islamist groups since the early 1990s, and for the conviction and imprisonment of thousands of political prisoners for their membership in such groups. Repression of alleged Islamist sympathizers increased after a bomb in Djerba in 2002 killed twenty-one people, followed by mass military trials of hundreds of presumed religious extremists. Tunisia is the only one of the three countries that does not have a legally recognized Islamist political party.

Morocco has also been criticized by international observers for the repression and imprisonment of alleged religious extremists after a series of simultaneous bombings in Casablanca killed over fifty people in May 2003. Suicide bombings in 2007, including one near the U.S. consulate, resulted in heightened anti-terror activity; Moroccan security actively pursue suspected terrorists, and the country has been on moderate to high anti-terror alert ever since.

After the Algerian government's cancellation of the 1992 parliamentary elections in which the Islamist Salvation Front Party was poised to win, Algeria went through a decade-long civil war between state security forces and armed Islamic groups, resulting in approximately 100,000 deaths and thousands of "disappeared" still unaccounted for. A national referendum was held in September 2005 on President Bouteflika's Charter for Peace and National Reconciliation, resulting in approval by an overwhelming majority. However, international and local human rights nongovernmental organizations (NGOs; see the glossary) denounced the referendum due to the considerable impunity the charter's amnesty plan accords to the state security forces, state armed militias, and armed Islamist groups. While officially the civil war has ended, security remains a concern in Algeria. The U.S. State Department has travel warnings in effect for travel to Algeria.

Current Issues Impacting Women's Rights to Health in the Maghreb

Women's status in the Maghreb, as it is worldwide, is characterized by inequality and discrimination, economic dependence, marginalization, and policies and attitudes that give control over women's bodies and sexual behavior to individual men, the family, and the state. Several factors common to all three countries affect women's abilities to access their human and legal rights.

One key factor is the role played by religion in issues related to women. Morocco, Algeria, and Tunisia have family codes or personal status laws governing marriage, divorce, child custody and guardianship, parentage, inheritance, and marital property—all based on the Maliki school of Islam. In all three countries, these are the only laws inspired by religious precepts, and they allow for large judicial discretion to interpret and apply Islamic jurisprudence and reasoning.[9] In contrast, legislation governing areas such as contracts, torts, criminal laws, administration, and commerce are based on secular, European-style civil codes. By removing family matters from the rule of law, this encourages resolving family disputes outside of the formal justice system. As an example, initiatives to promote and develop family mediation programs (to resolve what are legal disputes anywhere else) are increasingly popular among both governments and local NGOs.

Relatively high illiteracy rates among women and rural populations, and wide urban-rural disparities in the availability and proximity of such infrastructures as justice system personnel, education, and transportation impact women's ability to access their rights. Rural women are physically remote from public and private service providers. Women's illiteracy prevents them from knowing their legal rights and makes them vulnerable to misinformation and propaganda.

Women's rights and issues of sexuality are surrounded by a conservative legal, social, and religious context. Many issues have long been considered too sensitive to address openly and directly. However, several topics previously considered taboo in the Maghreb are now becoming increasingly more openly debated, popularized through the press and cultural media, integrated into local NGO programs, and even integrated into official speeches. Because of a hesitancy or lack of political will to tackle sensitive issues with concrete institutional and legal reforms, the family and criminal laws in the three countries have not caught up and do not effectively respond to current and changing economic circumstances and social realities.

Even existing laws and regulations that protect women's rights in theory are often not applied in practice. Authorities charged with enforcing the laws, such as the police and judges, frequently do not apply the laws properly, and in remote regions, there is no justice system infrastructure. As one rural health worker described to the chapter authors, "The law doesn't reach here because no one is coming to enforce it."

Family Laws

Tunisia has the reputation of having a particularly advanced Personal Status Code for the region. In contrast to the majority of Muslim legal systems, polygamy is illegal in Tunisia, both spouses have the right to initiate divorce on equal grounds, and husbands do not have the right to unilaterally repudiate their wife in an extrajudicial divorce without cause. However, discrimination against women continues to exist in property rights, unequal inheritance laws, and marital property laws that attribute property acquired during marriage to the husband in the absence of an optional community property contract. In addition, judges often decide cases on the basis of their interpretation of religious laws.

The Moroccan Family Code, promulgated in February 2004, contained major reforms impacting women: raising the age of marriage for women from fifteen to eighteen (the same as for men); placing the family under the joint responsibility of both spouses; rescinding the wife's duty of obedience to her husband; eliminating the requirement of a male marital tutor (*wali*) for women to marry; creating divorces by mutual consent and irreconcilable differences; placing polygamy and repudiation under judicial control; and creating the possibility for couples to sign a contract establishing joint marital property.

However, failure to apply the new laws by courts and in practice has been frequently documented. In reality, women often still have a *wali* conclude the marriage for them. A *wali*, often a woman's closest adult male relative, represents her in choosing a husband and conveys her consent to the marriage. In addition, the majority of men's petitions to take a second wife are still granted by courts. Despite the legal requirement that marriages be concluded with a written contract and registered with the authorities, in rural areas people are still getting married through traditional *ourfi* (oral) marriages, without the benefit of official documentation.

Increasing the minimum legal age of marriage from fifteen to eighteen has potential health benefits for women, including reduced health risks and decreased maternal mortality related to lower fertility rates and increased age at pregnancy. Later marriages can also contribute to a more equal balance of power within the marriage and enable women to have more control over decisions affecting their health.[10] However, raising the minimum legal age for marriage has been one of the most problematic reforms in terms of its consistent application. Under the law, the family affairs judge in charge of marriage may only authorize the marriage of a girl or boy under eighteen after conducting an enquiry that involves interviews with the parents, a social assessment, and medical expertise. The judge must issue a written decision justifying the marriage of a minor.[11] In reality, marriages of girls as young as thirteen and fourteen are still reported; the number of petitions for authorization to marry a minor girl increase each year; and the majority of these petitions are granted. In 2007, 87 percent of petitions to marry a girl under eighteen were granted, and marriages of minors comprised 10 percent of all marriages that year.[12]

The 1984 Algerian Family Code was likewise amended in February 2005 by presidential decree. The reforms did not go nearly as far as reforms in Morocco and were met with disappointment by women's groups. The law still discriminates against women in numerous ways, including the mandatory male marital tutor (*wali*) to sign marriage contracts on behalf of the bride, the impossibility for women to obtain divorce except

WOMEN'S ATTITUDES ABOUT IMPORTANT ISSUES IN THE MARRIAGE CONTRACT

Women in the Maghreb consider joint decision making on family planning a priority area in need of improvement in spousal relationships. In the fall of 2007, NGOs conducted community consultations in fifteen regions across Morocco, Algeria, and Tunisia, interviewing 1,474 women as part of an action-research project on the marriage contract. Women in twelve of the fifteen regions identified family planning as a topic they would like to include in their marriage contract to protect their rights.[17] Women's attitudes about including such issues as family planning or birth spacing in marriage contracts varied by age. The majority of younger women (thirty-eight and younger) felt that it was fundamental to agree in advance and negotiate clauses in the marriage contract about: spacing between pregnancies (they suggested three years); number of children; minimum amount of time between marriage and the first pregnancy (they suggested three years to make sure that the marriage would succeed before deciding to have children); and contraceptive use. Participants gave numerous examples of women whose forced successive pregnancies had a negative impact on their social and economic status. They described how some men use children as a way to pressure their wives to stay at home and not work outside; they told of women from their communities whose health suffered because of multiple pregnancies.

In contrast, participants age fifty and older objected to the stipulation of such conditions in the marriage contract for a number of reasons: arbitrary circumstances of life and destiny; the very personal nature of the topic makes it inappropriate for such intervention; and the idea that one should not interfere with God's will.

In addition, women in nine of the fifteen regions surveyed identified (spontaneously and without prompting) medical care as a right they would like to guarantee through a clause in their marriage contract.[18] Most participants, particularly those who were unemployed, asked for access to medical care in case they get sick, the right to preserve their health, a prohibition of remarriage by a husband whose first wife is sick,

and a ban on repudiation of women who are sterile or have a permanent illness. They wanted husbands to take care of wives when they are
sick and not send them back home to their families. They described how
even husbands who take care of their children's health do not provide
the same attention and care to their wives. In Tlemcen (Algeria), participants listened to the moving testimony of a woman with breast cancer
who, after being humiliated by her own family, was rejected and repudi-
ated by her husband, and left the conjugal home without receiving any
medical care.

The single most important issue cited by the women across the
three countries was domestic violence and cruelty. In all fifteen regions,
women uniformly proposed that a clause prohibiting all forms of violence—physical, sexual, psychological, and verbal—be a fundamental
condition for a marriage contract. Women described how they would
like to have marriages based on respect and dialogue. Participants gave
examples of violence they suffer in their own lives, from insults and of-
fences, to one wife's exploitation by her husband who forces her to go to
work and beats her when she comes back without any money.

for very specific reasons limited by the law, the persistence of polygamy,
and unequal inheritance rights for men and women.

In Algeria, many women's situations after divorce are exacerbated by
the country's severe housing crisis, particularly in Algiers, the capital.
The shortage of places to live, combined with the lack of alimony and
no division of marital property, means that women frequently end up
homeless after a divorce. While the 2005 Family Code reforms guarantee to women who have custody of their children the right to remain
in the conjugal home until the father provides adequate alternative
housing,[13] the law remains largely unenforced.

International observers in the region have expressed concerns that
women do not have the right to decide freely and responsibly about the
number, spacing, and timing of their children. Nor do they have the information and means to do so, or the right to attain the highest standard of sexual and reproductive health. This includes the right to make

decisions about reproduction free from discrimination, coercion, and violence.[14] It is interesting to note that the recently reformed Moroccan and Algerian Family Codes include consultation on decisions concerning family planning[15] and dialogue on the spacing of births[16] among the mutual rights and duties of spouses.

Sexual Relations outside of Marriage

Sexual relations outside of marriage are illegal in the Maghreb, with increased penalties in cases where one or both parties are married to another person. While all three countries' penal codes prohibit adultery,[19] only the Moroccan code explicitly prohibits sexual relations between unmarried single persons of the opposite sex.[20] In Morocco and Algeria, sexual relations between unmarried persons are considered a crime against morality; in Tunisia sexual relations between unmarried couples is considered a violation of the policy to ban the practice of unregistered *ourfi* or *fatiha* (verbal) marriages. These laws have both symbolic and real impacts; because sexual relations outside of marriage are defined as illicit, people are still imprisoned under these Penal Code provisions.

A recent survey suggests that such legal prohibitions have an impact on sexual education and safe sex practices: 68 percent of Moroccans have never received any sexual education; 32 percent think that sex education is harmful for children; 70 percent viewed sexual relations as motivated by the desire to have children; 28 percent considered sex to please the husband.[21]

Contraceptive use among young couples is low; one study suggests that less than half of young couples in Morocco use any form of contraception.[22] Official government policy treats contraception as a family planning method to space pregnancies only within the context of marriage, and not as a form of birth control for unmarried couples. The morning-after pill was made available for sale in Morocco in 2008, nearly ten years after the first pharmaceutical application to market the pill in 1999. Marketed as a preventive method for married couples only in the context of healthy family planning, the pill is supposed to be available only with a doctor's prescription, but pharmacies frequently sell it without a prescription. However, pharmacists often refuse to provide guidance or instructions for its use, leaving consumers on their own to read the written instructions—printed in English and French, but not Arabic. In addition, the price of the morning after pill — 92 *dirhams* (about $11) — is too expensive for many women.

In Tunisia, family planning programs have been designed and implemented as part of a larger national economic development strategy, rather than as part of a rights-based approach to women's health and sexuality. Ever since independence, Tunisia's health strategy has paid particular attention to women because of the impact of reproduction on demographics and population. The importation and sale of contraceptives has been authorized in Tunisia since 1961, although the official government stance links contraception with the desire to space pregnancies within marriage and to not procreate unless there is the desire to have children — always within marriage.[23]

Virginity

The legal prohibition of sexual relations outside of marriage and the importance placed on female "intactness" before marriage, combined with the increasing number of single people in their late twenties and thirties and changing social norms, lead to contradictory behaviors and attitudes about female virginity. There is no similar cultural or social imperative for men to remain virgins before marriage.

Today's Moroccan magazines contain numerous articles discussing virginity, the extent to which it is still important for women to be virgins upon marriage, and attempts to assess the reality. Several articles — quite audacious in their reporting — denounce what they characterize as the societal hypocrisy of current laws, perceived as contradictory to and out of touch with reality. Sexual relations prior to marriage are becoming more and more frequent, according to these articles. While an increasing number of women may lose their virginity before marriage, the idea that a woman will be lucky to find a man who will "accept them as they are," "despite their handicap" is still prevalent, and the attitude among men is frequently that they are disappointed but they will *forgive* the woman. Often girls may give in to their boyfriends' advances upon promises of marriage.[24] The common interpretation in the media is that only a minority of young women are having sexual relations prior to marriage, and that these women are mainly from the relatively well-off urban elite.[25] However, people's hesitation to speak openly about their own experiences makes it difficult to get an accurate picture of this phenomenon.

"Arriving intact" at one's marriage is still a strong social imperative in Morocco. Practices such as obtaining virginity certificates or having an operation to restore one's hymen illustrate the extent to which young women are prepared to go to preserve appearances. Operations in private urban clinics in Morocco to restore a hymen can cost 2,000–3,000 *dirhams* ($250–$350). One gynecologist, originally opposed to practicing hymen reconstructive surgery, describes her change of mind in order to treat the "psychological suffering" of women who fear they will not be able to get married because they are no longer virgins.[26] Even couples who themselves know that the woman is not a virgin may resort to using animal blood or cutting themselves on the wedding night to provide "evidence" that the woman was a virgin.

Perceived or real pressure from families can play a large role in a couple's relationship. One survey reported that 62 percent of young Moroccans think that having a premarital sexual relationship would be complicated, with the major obstacles being the family and the neighbors. As one woman described it, "When I announced to my boyfriend—who considered himself open-minded—that I was not a virgin, he turned blue and exclaimed, 'what will I tell my mother?' "[27] There exists a kind of cultural schizophrenia and contradictory societal imperatives related to female sexuality. In a sense, many young women in the Maghreb feel that no matter what they do it will be wrong, and will make them vulnerable to public criticism and judgment.

Abortion

Both the Moroccan and Algerian penal codes criminalize abortion under legal provisions found in the section of the law on crimes and misdemeanors against public morality.[28] Abortion is illegal unless deemed necessary to protect the mother's health (Morocco) or to protect the mother's life (Algeria), and in both countries it must be performed by a medical doctor.[29] In Morocco, an abortion may be performed only within the first six weeks of pregnancy, and the husband's authorization is required, except in cases where the mother's life is in danger. In the absence of spousal authorization, the doctor must seek written permission from the chief medical doctor in the district before performing the abortion.[30] Algerian and Moroccan laws punish a woman who has an abortion (or attempts to have one) for reasons other than maternal life or health,[31] as well as anyone who is deemed to have incited an abortion through public statements or the distribution of written or visual materials.[32] In contrast, abortion was legalized in Tunisia in 1965, where it must be performed by a medical doctor within the first three months of pregnancy. Tunisian law does not require the woman to provide a reason for seeking an abortion or the husband's authorization.[33]

Despite highly restrictive laws in Algeria and Morocco, the few studies that have been conducted on abortion suggest a very high incidence rate in the two countries. An estimated 600 women have an abortion in Morocco each day. According to the World Health Organization (WHO; see the glossary), 13 percent of maternal mortality in North African countries is due to unsafe abortion.[34] This would mean that in Morocco there are 219,000 illegal abortions per year, and 600,000 births. Police may be alerted when women are admitted in critical condition to public hospitals for complications related to illegal abortions. This situation no doubt dissuades women from seeking medical care when they need it after an abortion, out of fear of arrest.

A campaign to change this situation is being led by the Association Marocaine de Lutte contre l'Avortement Clandestin (Moroccan Association against Clandestine Abortion, MACA), an NGO that lobbies for reforms to the abortion law to allow abortion in cases of rape, incest, fetal malformations, or psychiatric disorders of the mother, and to eliminate clandestine, unsafe abortions. The chief doctor at a leading Rabat public hospital maternity ward founded MACA because of his alarm at the number of women admitted to the hospital with complications related to clandestine abortion. He was also concerned about children abandoned shortly after birth, suicide attempts by young pregnant women, and the eviction of unmarried pregnant women from their family homes. This relatively bold organization is attempting to break the taboo on abortion in Morocco not by calling for a complete liberalization of the laws, but by enlarging the criteria for therapeutic abortion (in French, an *interruption médicale de grossesse*, or IMG), and by distinguishing between a therapeutic abortion and a "social" abortion (an *interruption volontaire de grossesse*, or IVG). The association's arguments are grounded in a public health perspective and not a rights-based approach.[35]

It is estimated that such a liberalization of the abortion laws would eliminate the need for huge numbers of nonmedical and clandestine abortions and reduce the cost of an abortion from the current 2,000–10,000 Moroccan *dirhams* ($235–$1,175 for an illicit operation) to 1,000 *dirhams* ($118). The Moroccan media reflect the society's ambivalence on this issue; comments range from congratulatory to the association for trying to break the taboo on the topic, contrasting the high rate of abortion in Morocco to the lower rates in countries where abortion is legal, to calls for the association's members to submit to Allah, and pronouncements that abortion is against Islam.

Violence against Women

Violence against women in the Maghreb is considered a private matter and is significantly underreported, uninvestigated by law enforcement, and unpunished by the judicial systems. There are many factors that contribute to this pattern: beliefs—supported by religion—that there are circumstances that justify wife battering; fear and shame on the part of victims; social stigma; the lack of legal protection for women under current laws; women's lack of awareness of their legal rights that do exist, or lack of faith in the justice system, or inability to afford legal representation at court proceedings; and the conservative, sometimes insensitive, attitudes of law enforcement officers and justice system personnel.

None of the three Maghreb countries has specific violence-against-women legislation. Domestic and other forms of violence against women are covered under generally applicable homicide and assault and battery provisions in the penal codes. The existing laws in the Maghreb are insufficient to prevent, investigate, and punish domestic and other forms of gender-based violence—and the few existing laws are seldom enforced by the police or the courts. There are no civil remedies for protection and compensation of female victims of violence, such as civil protection or temporary restraining orders, mechanisms for ordering the violent offender out of the home, or provisions related to divorce proceedings, property use, financial maintenance during separation, or compensatory damages.

Both under the law and in practice, victims of violence need an actual injury to prove assault and battery. Existing laws address only serious physical violence, and they focus on the results of the acts rather than the offender's behavior. Sliding-scale sentences are determined by the severity of consequences, requiring a victim in Morocco to provide a doctor's certificate of a disability lasting at least twenty days[36] or proof of a permanent disability resulting from the violence. Courts rarely punish offenders for less than the threshold disability or for "low level" misdemeanor violence (slaps, scratches, threats, and insults) common in domestic violence. In addition, the current laws in all three countries only cover physical violence, and do not include psychological, verbal, emotional, or economic violence.

In Morocco, the Criminal Procedure Code allows "proof by any means," but in practice the courts do not find an offender guilty without medical certificates, witnesses, and photos in cases of domestic violence. Thus, proving domestic assault and battery is quite difficult. Women's groups in several regions in Morocco have successfully lobbied the local health ministry delegations to provide free medical certificates to female victims of violence at local hospitals. However, it can be difficult to get the police to respond to a domestic violence complaint. The widely repeated comment is that when one calls the police in domestic assault cases, the first question they ask is *"Wash kayn el dim?"* ("Is there blood?")—because if there is not, the likelihood of getting a quick police response, if any at all, is quite low.

The Moroccan Penal Code has provisions that pose problems for protecting women from domestic violence. Harboring a married woman who has left the conjugal home without her husband's consent is a criminal offense. As a result family, friends, and NGOs technically can be prosecuted for sheltering an abused woman who has fled a violent husband—which is the answer to the question often asked by foreign observers, "Why are there no shelters for women victims of violence in Morocco?"[37]

Family laws also impact the rights of women who are victims of domestic violence. The 2004 Moroccan Family Code eliminated the wife's duty of obedience to her husband, but the Penal Code still maintains the concept of the husband's legal "authority" over the wife. Under the Family Code, a wife who flees the conjugal home and refuses to return when ordered to do so by the court loses her right to financial maintenance from her husband. While the Family Code introduced divorce for irreconcilable differences, a wife still has the right to petition for a fault-based divorce because of harm. However, the lack of a specific definition of harm, difficulty in proving it, the length of fault-based divorce proceedings, and judicial resistance are all reasons why the majority of divorce petitions in domestic violence cases are filed as or converted to irreconcilable differences cases, resulting in the abused wife's loss of many of her rights. In Algeria, the severe economic consequences of divorce and the housing crisis may compel women to stay in a violent marriage for lack of other options.

Conjugal violence is the most frequent form of violence against women in Algeria,[38] although gender-based violence has been exacerbated due to the country's decade-long internal armed conflict, in which women were victims of violence (abduction, rape, and murder) perpetrated by armed Islamist groups, civilian militias, and state security forces.[39] The disappearance of men during the conflict has caused numerous legal and administrative difficulties for their wives. Under the Algerian Family Code, men are the legal tutors (guardians) of their children unless the court rules that they are dead or missing; wives need such a ruling in order to be able to sign legal and administrative documents for their children. Also, women are left with no access to bank accounts, property registered in their missing husband's name, pensions, or other social benefits. Obtaining a death certificate for men abducted and presumed killed by Islamist groups can take years.[40]

It is worth noting that the Penal Codes in all three countries treat rape as a crime against morality (thus creating an inappropriate link between rape and illicit sexual relations). The laws do not define rape clearly, nor do they include any clear directives as to evidence collection and standards of proof in rape cases.[41] Non-consent is difficult for victims to prove, often requiring evidence of actual physical injury. If rape is not proven, charges may then be brought against the victim for having engaged in illicit sexual relations. In Morocco, the penalties for rape are the same as those for indecent assault, with rape of a virgin victim or of a pregnant woman considered an aggravating circumstance. Criminal proceedings against rapists of underage girls can be cancelled if the offender marries his victim, and marital rape is not a criminal offense in the Penal Code (despite the new Family Law's elimination of the wife's duty of obedience to her husband).

Over the past several years, women's rights NGOs in large cities across the Maghreb have begun to address the issue of violence against women by opening *centres d'écoute* (counseling centers) for women victims of violence. These centers have succeeded in breaking the taboo surrounding violence against women. To date, the activities of these centers, international organizations, and the national governments have been limited to individual counseling for women and public awareness-raising campaigns to draw attention to the existence of violence against women. They have not focused on enacting legal reforms to address the problem.

Violence against women is a major problem—particularly domestic violence, sexual harassment, and rape. However, it remains widely hidden and underreported. Data from NGO counseling centers in Morocco indicate that in nine out of ten cases of violence against women, the assailants are men with whom the victims have had an intimate relationship; in eight out of ten cases, the perpetrator is the husband.[42] In the first half of 2007, there were 16,527 official complaints of gender-based physical and sexual violence filed in Morocco. In cases examined from six courts across Morocco, 32 percent of cases related to women's rights concerned issues of physical violence.[43]

The most recent Moroccan report to the UN Committee on the Elimination of Discrimination against Women (CEDAW)—set up by a 1979 treaty that bans gender discrimination—notes tentative steps taken by the government to address violence against women: awareness-raising campaigns; the opening of two specialized hospital centers in Rabat and Casablanca to address violence against women; the creation of special interagency focal points at the local level for women victims of violence; and the establishment of a national hotline for women victims of violence.[44]

International treaty-monitoring bodies have found that the three countries have not met their obligations to address violence against women. CEDAW has told all three countries that violence-against-women legislation is necessary in order for them to be in compliance with international obligations, and they have been urged to draft such legislation as a matter of urgency.[45] The Moroccan government has for several years declared its intention to promulgate such legislation. In November 2006, then Moroccan Prime Minister Driss Jettou announced a national campaign on violence against women. Since then the government has issued public statements that a draft bill on violence against women is forthcoming, although none has yet been presented.

Local NGO Work and International Presence in the Maghreb

Compared to other countries in the Maghreb, there are comparatively few international or nongovernmental organizations working on humanitarian, development, or women's rights issues in Tunisia. This may be due to both the perception that Tunisia is more "advanced" in these areas than other countries in the region and hence less in need, and to the difficulties of working in a strongly government-controlled context. The state in Tunisia tends to appropriate local development and human rights issues as part of its own agenda, to the exclusion of independent initiatives. Thus, the government maintains an extremely tight rein on independent NGOs, especially those working on human rights issues. While there are thousands of local associations in towns and villages across the country, the majority of these are considered state-sponsored, with only a handful of truly autonomous local human and women's rights NGOs. International workers may have difficulties working in Tunisia, which requires government authorization for all activities and is highly restrictive. Representatives of the international NGO Reporters without Borders have been barred from entering the country, and both UN and international NGO employees report having had their bags searched and publications and documents confiscated by the customs police upon arrival at the airport. In addition to the practical challenges of working in this system, it is difficult to form the healthy interpersonal relationships conducive to effective work under such circumstances.

In contrast, there are a growing number of autonomous NGOs throughout Algeria addressing a diversity of issues including women's and human rights, Amazigh rights, the disappeared, and local development. Algeria had more than a decade of isolation from the international community during its civil war, but international organizations have now begun to launch programs in the country, working particularly on democracy and human rights issues. The National Democratic Institute (which aims to strengthen democratic institutions worldwide), has worked in Algeria since 1997; Global Rights launched programs in Algeria from its Morocco office in 2003; the AFL-CIO Solidarity Center set up its Maghreb program from an Algiers-based regional office in 2006; and Médecins du Monde (Doctors of the World) opened an Algerian office in 2007. However, burdensome administrative procedures and governmental suspicion of outsiders and international NGOs in general can substantially delay initiatives.

There is a substantial international presence in Morocco, as the country has a long history of development cooperation with foreign actors. The U.S. Agency for International Development (USAID; see the glossary) has been present in Morocco for over fifty years, and the Peace Corps has been in Morocco since 1963. The local NGO movement in Morocco is quite dynamic, with human rights and women's rights NGOS and local development associations having proliferated in number and developed beyond the Rabat-Casablanca corridor over the last decade. There is a large number and wide diversity of private and public donors supporting civil society initiatives in Morocco. Many UN, international governmental, and NGO agencies run their Maghreb operations from Morocco-based offices due to the relative ease and freedom to operate there, as compared to other countries in the region.

Conclusion

Wide diversity across communities in the Maghreb creates the imperative for multifaceted programs to address the people's varied circumstances. For example, an organization that develops a human rights education program for women that depends heavily on written materials will be censored for contributing to a two-track development process that excludes those who are illiterate. Authenticity is sometimes used as a synonym for traditions. It may be invoked to rationalize what seem to be discriminatory practices and as a justification to resist politically and socially sensitive change. Modernity may be used to counter the fact that marginalization and underdevelopment still exist in many communities, or to defend against perceived accusations of backwardness. For example, illustrated materials depicting women in traditional dress or in rural areas may be met with official reactions of "that is not the real Moroccan (or Algerian or Tunisian) woman," countered with examples of the number of female pilots, doctors, or government ministers the country has. Finally, local specificities are frequently cited to foreigners as the reason why models and examples from other countries may not be workable or appropriate in the country.

Travelers to the Maghreb should keep in mind these frequently cited concepts as they participate in international development and exchange projects in the region. The regional approach of this chapter illustrates how different attitudes and solutions are often applied to similar circumstances. Cross-fertilization and sharing of strategies across the Maghreb are encouraged, as they help both international and local actors identify and evolve future best practices for the region.

Millennium Development Goal indicators are italicized.

TABLE 5.1 : **POPULATION AND HUMAN DEVELOPMENT**

	Algeria	Morocco	Tunisia
POPULATION			
Total	34.178 million	34.859 million	10.486 million
Population growth rate	1.2%	1.48%	0.98%
Net migration rate/1,000 population	−0.29	−0.72	−0.41
Urban	65%	56%	67%
Rural	35%	44%	33%
AGE STRUCTURE			
0–14 years	25.4%	30%	22.7%
15–64 years	69.5%	64.7%	70.1%
65+ years	5.1%	5.2%	7.2%
Median age (years)	26.6	25.0	29.2
MAJOR ETHNIC GROUPS			
Arab/Amizigh	99%	99.1%	98%
European/Jewish	< 1%	0.9%	2%
RELIGIONS			
Sunni Muslim	99%	98.7%	98%
Christian and Jewish	1%	1.3%	2%
HUMAN DEVELOPMENT			
Human Development Index	0.748	0.646	0.762
Human Development rank[a]	100th	127th	95th
Freedom House Index	Not free	Part free	Not free
Political Rights score[b]	6	5	7
Civil Liberties score[b]	5	4	5
Human Poverty Index	21.5%	33.4%	17.9%
Human Poverty rank[c]	104th	126th	91st

Notes: [a]out of 179 countries; [b]1 = most free, 7 = least free; [c]out of 177 countries

TABLE 5.2 : **GOVERNMENT AND ECONOMY**

	Algeria	Morocco	Tunisia
GOVERNMENT			
Independence	5 Jul. 1962 from France	2 Mar. 1956 from France	20 Mar. 1956 from France
Type of government	Republic	Constitutional monarchy	Republic
Voting rights	Age 18, universal	Age 18, universal	Age 18, universal
CAPITAL	Algiers	Rabat	Tunis
CURRENCY	Algerian dinars (DZD)	Moroccan dirhams (MAD)	Tunisian dinars (TND)
ECONOMY			
Gross domestic product (GDP) (in PPP US $)	232.9 billion	136.6 billion	81.71 billion
Annual GDP growth	NA	4.9%	NA
GDP per capita (in US $)	$6,900	$4,700	$7,900
Gini Index	35.3	40	40
Population living below PPP $1/day	7.0%	2.5%	2.6%
External debt	$2.7 billion	$21.22 billion	$20.81 billion
Public debt as % of GDP	9.9	59.7	48.4
Official development assistance (ODA) per capita (in US $)	$11.1	$21.6	$37.6
Foreign direct investment as % of GDP	NA	NA	NA
LABOR FORCE			
In agriculture	14%	44.6%	55%
In industry	13.4%	19.8%	23%
In services	24.6%	35.5%	22%
Other	48% (32% of which is in government)	NA	NA
Unemployment rate	12.5%	10%	14.1%

TABLE 5.3 : **GEOGRAPHY AND ENVIRONMENT**

	Algeria	Morocco	Tunisia
LAND COMPOSITION			
Land area	2,381,741 sq. km. (918,923 sq. mi.)	446,550 sq. km. (172,443 sq. mi.)	163,610 sq. km. (63,166 sq. mi.)
Size comparison	Slightly less than 3 times Texas	Slightly larger than California	Slightly larger than Georgia
Terrain	Mostly high plateau and desert; some mountains; coastal plain; 988-km. (614-mi.) coastline on Mediterranean Sea	Mountainous coast and interior; plateaus, valleys, rich coastal plain; 1,835-km. (1,140-mi.) coastline on Atlantic Ocean and Mediterranean	Mountains; hot, dry central plain; semi-arid south merges into Sahara; 1,148-km. (413-mi.) coastline on Mediterranean
Ecological hazards	Earthquakes in mountainous areas, mudslides and floods in rainy season	Earthquakes in northern mountains, periodic droughts	NA
LAND USE AND RESOURCES			
Permanent crop land	0.28%	2%	13.08%
Arable land	3.17%	19%	17.05%
Agricultural products	Wheat, barley, oats, grapes, olives, citrus, fruit, livestock	Barley, wheat, citrus, wine, vegetables, olives, livestock	Olives, olive oil, grain, citrus, tomatoes, beef, dairy, sugar
Natural resources	Petroleum, natural gas, iron ore, phosphates, uranium, lead, zinc	Phosphates, iron ore, manganese, lead, zinc, fish, salt	Petroleum, salt, phosphate, iron ore, lead, zinc
ENVIRONMENTAL ISSUES	Soil erosion from overgrazing and poor farming techniques; desertification; pollution of rivers and coastal waters; inadequate supplies of potable water	Land degradation and desertification; raw sewage contamination of water supplies; oil pollution of coastal waters	Hazards from toxic waste disposal; raw sewage water pollution; overgrazing, deforestation, and desertification
INFRASTRUCTURE			
Population with access to improved water source	85%	83%	94%
Population using improved sanitation	94%	72%	85%
Roadways unpaved	29.8%	38.1%	34.2%

TABLE 5.4 : **HEALTH**

	Algeria	Morocco	Tunisia
LIFE, BIRTH, DEATH			
Life expectancy at birth (male/female)	72.3/75.7	69.4/74.3	73.9/77.7
Birth rate/1,000 population	16.9	20.9	15.4
Death rate/1,000 population	4.6	5.45	5.2
Infant mortality rate/1,000 live births	*33.0*	*32.0*	*22.5*
PERSONNEL AND INFRASTRUCTURE			
Physicians/100,000 population	110	51	134
Hospital beds/10,000 population	21	8	17
HEALTH ECONOMICS			
Total expenditure on health per capita (PPP US $)	$315	$207	$355
Public expenditure on health as % of GDP	4.2	5.3	5.1
DISEASES			
Most common vector-borne diseases	NA	NA	NA
Most common food- and water-borne diseases	Bacterial diarrhea, hepatitis A, typhoid fever	Bacterial diarrhea, hepatitis A	Bacterial diarrhea, hepatitis A
TB incidence/100,000 pop.	*56.6*	*91.6*	*26.0*
TB prevalence/100,000 pop.	*55.9*	*79.9*	*28.4*
New TB cases HIV-positive	0.6%	0.5%	1.3%
New TB cases multidrug-resistant (MDR)	1.2%	0.5%	2.6%
1-year-olds fully immunized against TB	99%	96%	99%
Estimated malaria cases annually	NA	NA	NA
Malaria death rate/100,000 population	NA	NA	NA
HIV prevalence rate in adults	*0.1%*	*0.1%*	*< 0.1%*
AIDS deaths in adults annually	*< 1,000*	*< 1,000*	*< 200*
People living with HIV	21,000	21,000	3,700
AIDS orphans	NA	NA	NA

Fertility rate (children born per woman)	1.79	2.51	1.72
Contraceptive prevalence rate (married women 15–49)	*61%*	*63%*	*66%*
Maternal mortality rate/100,000 births	*180*	*240*	*100*
Lifetime risk of maternal death, 1 in:	*220*	*150*	*500*
Births attended by skilled birth attendant	*95%*	*63%*	*90%*
CHILD HEALTH			
Mortality rate of children < 5/1,000 live births	*37*	*34*	*21*
1-year-olds immunized against measles	*92%*	*95%*	*98%*
Children < 5 using insecticide-treated bed nets	*NA*	*NA*	*NA*
Children < 5 with fever treated with antimalarial drugs	*NA*	*NA*	*NA*
Newborns protected against tetanus	70%	85%	96%
HUNGER AND MALNUTRITION			
Children < 5 underweight for age	*4.3%*	*12.2%*	*4.6%*
Children < 5 under height for age	*NA*	*10%*	*NA*
Population undernourished	*5.0%*	*5.0%*	*5.0%*

TABLE 5.5 : **LANGUAGE, EDUCATION, AND LITERACY**

	Algeria	Morocco	Tunisia
LANGUAGES			
Arabic, French, Tamazight dialects	A. (official), Fr., and Tamazight	A. (official), Fr. (lang. of business, government, diplomacy)	A. (official), Fr. (lang. of commerce)
LITERACY			
Adult literacy rate (population age 15+ who can read and write)	69.9%	52.3%	74.3%
EXPENDITURE			
Public expenditure on education as % of GDP	5.1	NA	7.3
Net enrollment in primary education[d]	96.0%	89.3%	96.6%
School life expectancy, in years (male/female)[e]	13/13	11/9	13/14

[d]Net enrollment rate in primary education is measured as the number of children of official primary school age who are enrolled in primary education as a percentage of children in the official primary school age population.

[e]School life expectancy is the total number of years of school (from primary through tertiary education) that a child can expect to receive.

Principal Sources for Data in Appendix Tables 5.1–5.5

Central Intelligence Agency, *The World Factbook* (https://www.cia.gov/library/publications/the-world-factbook/).

UNDP Human Development Report, 2007/2008, available at: www.hdrstats.undp.org.

UN Millennium Development Goals Indicators Database, available at www.mdgs.un.org.

UNICEF. The State of the World's Children 2009. Available at http://www.data.un.org.

NOTES

The authors thank Houda Benmbarek for her research assistance for this chapter. We also thank the numerous Peace Corps volunteers, Fulbright scholars, representatives of local nongovernmental organizations, and lawyers from all three countries in the Maghreb who kindly agreed to be interviewed for this chapter.

1. As one observer commented to one of the chapter authors, "Algeria is a rich country that is very poor, because its oil revenue is not widely distributed among the population or used to finance internal development."

2. Tamazight is the correct name for the language commonly referred to as Berber, and Amazigh is the name used for the people who speak the language.

3. The United Nations Committee on the Elimination of Racial Discrimination has on several occasions criticized Tunisia's government for its position toward the Amazigh population, for example, for failing to enact legislation to protect against racial discrimination of the Amazigh and assuring their rights to cultural and language preservation. See, for example, Office of the United Nations High Commissioner for Human Rights, Committee on the Elimination of Racial Discrimination, 74th Session, 16 February–6 March 2009 (www.imadr.org/un/CERD74rpt_final.pdf). Also see http://www.buzzle.com/articles/unesco-devastating-report-on-anti-berber-racial-discrimination-in-tunisia.html.

4. Specifically, the Moroccan Ministry of Habous and Islamic Affairs, the Algerian Ministry of Religious Affairs and Wakfs, and the Tunisian Ministry of Religious Affairs.

5. The five pillars are: professing the unity of God and Mohammed's role as his Prophet; saying the five daily prayers; giving alms; fasting during Ramadan; and making a pilgrimage to Mecca.

6. In Morocco and Tunisia, the weekend falls on Saturday and Sunday; in Algeria, it falls on Thursday and Friday.

7. The current Moroccan minister of social development, the family, and solidarity was the subject of polemics in the media in the spring of 2008 for allegedly suggesting that the loudspeaker volume for the call to prayer should be reduced in order to avoid disturbing hospital patients and non-Muslims (interpreted in the press as "tourists").

8. In Tunisia, the sale of alcohol is prohibited every Friday (the holy day), while in Morocco, the sale of alcohol is suspended only on religious holidays. While not forbidden in Algeria, the sale of alcohol—usually available only in expensive hotels and restaurants—is not encouraged and is strictly monitored.

9. The laws are the Moroccan Personal Status Code, or Moudawana, which was the object of reforms in February 2004; the Algerian Family Code of 1984, modified in February 2005; and the Tunisian Personal Status Code of 1956, amended in 1992.

10. "Adding Health to the Discourse on the Moroccan Family Code: The Potential Women's Health Benefits Derived from an Increase in the Minimum Age of Marriage," Fulbright Scholar Working Paper. Washington, D.C.: The Fulbright Program. Council for International Exchange of Scholars, 2006.

11. Moroccan Family Code, article 20.

12. Ligue Democratique des droits des femmes/Democratic League for

Women's Rights. 4ᵉRapport Annuel,/Fourth Annual Report). Casablanca, Morocco, 2007.

13. Algerian Family Code, article 72.

14. "Violence against Women in Morocco." Prepared by Carin Benninger-Budel. The World Organisation Against Torture. For the Committee on the Elimination of Discrimination against Women. Presented at CEDAW's 29th session. New York, NY, 30 June-18 July 2003.

15. Moroccan Family Code, article 51.

16. Algerian Family Code, article 36.

17. See the website of Global Rights Maghreb (http://globalrightsmaghreb .files.wordpress.com) for more information on this program and its publications.

18. This right was not included in the project's protocol, nor was it on the list of topics provided to facilitators to be suggested to participants; it was raised by the women themselves. The nine regions include all five regions in Algeria where the consultations were held.

19. Article 491 of the Moroccan Penal Code punishes adultery with one to two years in prison, as does article 339 of the Algerian Penal Code, as amended in 1982. Article 236 of the Tunisian Penal Code, as modified in 1968, punishes adultery with a five-year prison sentence.

20. Article 490 of the Moroccan Penal Code punishes sexual relations between unmarried persons of the opposite sex with a prison sentence of one month to one year. Article 489 punishes immodest acts or acts against nature with persons of the same sex with six months to three years in prison.

21. "Virginité. Est-ce encore un tabou? Tel Quel, July 28, 2007, Telquel On-Line (http://www.telquel-online.com/284/couverture_284.shtml).

22. Jaouad Mdidech,"Relations sexuelles avant le mariage, les jeunes en parlent, " *La Vie Eco*, 6 May 2007 (http://www.bladi.net/12617-relations-sexuelles-mariage jeunes.html).

23. Les Femmes en Tunisie 2000 [in French] Tunis, Tunisia: Centre de Recherche, d' Etudes, de Documentation et d'Information sur la Femme, CREDIF. (2002; http://www.credif.org.tn/index.php?option=com_content&view=article &id=146&itemid=173&lang=fr).

24. Mdidech, "Relations sexuelles avant le mariage."

25. We are not convinced that is correct. Decades of anecdotal evidence and experience in diverse urban and rural areas suggest that even years ago, young couples in rural and smaller towns perceived as conservative were having sexual relations outside of marriage. It is possible that only now are urban dwellers starting to speak frankly about things they have been doing for years. It is also possible that the perception that young women are more sexually active now may be based on other, newer social phenomena (like the increasing number of

women in the workforce, and the greater number of restaurants and nightclubs frequented by young women), rather than on an actual increase in sexual relations before marriage among young women.

26. Habibou Bangré, "Maroc: réparer les hymens en secret," [Secret hymen repair in Morocco] 1 May 2009 (http://www.afriknews.com/article15639.html).

27. Ibid.

28. In Morocco, abortion is covered by articles 449-58 of the Penal Code, in the section on "Crimes and Misdemeanors against Family Order and Public Morality," as promulgated in 1962, with a few of the provisions on abortion last amended in 1967. In Algeria, abortion is covered in articles 304-310 of the Penal Code.

29. Articles 449-52 of the Moroccan Penal Code punish performing an abortion — unless it is required for the mother's health — with one to five years in prison (the sentence is doubled if the person performing the abortion habitually performs the procedure), and convicted medical professionals may also be barred from exercising their profession temporarily or permanently. The exemption to preserve the mother's life is in article 308 of the Algerian Penal Code. Articles 304-7 give the same punishment for performing other abortions as the Moroccan Penal Code articles above.

30. Moroccan Penal Code, article 453.

31. Article 454 of the Moroccan Penal Code and article 309 of the Algerian Penal Code both provide for a prison term of six months to two years for a woman who has or attempts to have an abortion.

32. Article 455 of the Moroccan Penal Code punishes a host of such acts with imprisonment for two months to two years, while article 310 of the Algerian Penal Code punishes these acts with a sentence of two months to three years.

33. Les Femmes en Tunisie 2000 [in French] Tunis, Tunisia: Centre de Recherche, d' Etudes, de Documentation et d'Information sur la Femme, CREDIF. (2002. http://www.credif.org.tn/index.php?option=com_content&view=article&id=146&itemid=173&lang=fr.

34. World Health Organization. Unsafe Abortion: Global and Regional Estimates of the Incidence of Unsafe Abortion and Associated Mortality. Geneva: WHO, 2004.

35. "L'homme qui veut légaliser l'avortement au Maroc," [The man who wants to legalize abortion in Morocco. In French] *Le Reporter*, 2 November 2008.

36. Algerian Penal Code provisions have a threshold of fifteen days' incapacity for any assault and battery complaint to be taken seriously by the justice system.

37. One of the authors of this chapter has heard reports of at least three residential shelters for female victims of violence in Morocco, but this is no more than hearsay, and the shelters' locations are kept secret.

38. *Livre Blanc: Violences contre les femmes et les enfants*, Algeria: Réseau Wassila, 2002).

39. The international humanitarian organization Médecins du Monde opened an office in Algeria in 2007 and works to reduce violence against women, mainly through support to the national hotline for victims of violence, training of local authorities and health personnel, and raising Algerians' awareness of the problem.

40. Amnesty International,"Algeria: Briefing to the Committee on the Elimination of Discrimination against Women," 1 December 2004. (http://www.amnesty.org/en/library/info/MDE28/011/2004).

41. See article 336 of the Algerian Penal Code, article 227 of the Tunisian Penal Code, and articles 486–88 of the Moroccan Penal Code.

42. See, for example, Ligue démocratique des droits des femmes, (The Democratic League of Women's Rights) "3e Rapport Annuel" Casablanca, Morocco, September 2006), and Anaruz Réseau National des Centres d'Ecoute des Femmes Victimes de Violences, "Les violences fondées sur le genre au Maroc: deuxième rapport" (2007).

43. Ligue démocratique des droits des femmes, "3e Rapport Annuel."

44. Ligue démocratique des droits des femmes, 3e Rapport Annuel, September 2006, and 4e Rapport Annuel, September 2007. Casablanca, Morocco.

45. Committee on the Elimination of Discrimination Against Women, CEDAW "Concluding Comments: Morocco," Geneva, Switzerland (24 January 2008), CEDAW "Concluding Comments: Algeria" Geneva, Switzerland (28 January 2005) http://www.unhchr.ch/tbs/doc.nsf/%28Symbol%29/A.60.38 (paras.129–167.en?opendocument), and CEDAW "Concluding Comments: Tunisia" (21 June 2002) http://www.unhchr.ch/tbs/doc.nsf/%28Symbol%29/A.57.38 ,paras.171%e2%80%93210.en?opendocument).

SUGGESTED WEBSITES

Algeria
Ministry of Health, http://www.sante.dz/.
Ministry of Justice, http://www.mjustice.dz/.
Ministry of State Charged with the Family and the Status of Women, http://www.ministere-famille.gov.dz.

Morocco
Ministry of Health, http://srvweb.sante.gov.ma/Pages/default.aspx.
Ministry of Justice, http://www.justice.gov.ma/index_fr.aspx.

Tunisia
Ministry of Health, http://www.santetunisie.rns.tn/msp/msp.html.
Tunisia Online News. http://tunisiaonlinenews.com/.

Femmes Tunisiennes (Tunisian Women): http://www.femmes.tn/eng/index2
.php?option+com_content&task=view&id=25&pop=1&page=6&itemid=42.

Other

Amazigh World [an organization that maintains a website providing current
information on news, human rights issues, music and culture, and history of
the Amizigh], http://www.amazighworld.org/.

Association AIDS Algérie (Algeria), http://www.aidsalgerie.org/.

Association de lutte contre le sida/Association for the fight against AIDS
(Morocco), http://www.alcsmaroc.ma/.

Le réseau Amazigh pour la citoynneté/The Amizigh network for citizenship
[an organization lobbying for Amazigh rights; its website provides information about Amazigh history and culture in the Maghreb], http://www
.reseauamazigh.org.

Tanmia (the National Human Resource Development and Employment Authority) provides training, career guidance, employment skills, and matches job
seekers and employers; it has regional offices across the United Arab Emir-
ates); http://www.tanmia.ma.

ADDENDUM: TUNISIA

The situation in Tunisia changed dramatically in late 2010 and early 2011, when
unprecedented popular protests took place, leading to a nationwide uprising.
Curfews and later a state of emergency were declared. The Internet played a crucial role in the movement, as Tunisians actively communicated breaking news,
photos and videos of events, and their own reactions through Facebook, Twitter,
and YouTube.

In mid-January, President Zine El Abidine Ben Ali and his family were forced to
flee the country. Prime Minister Mohammed Ghannouchi announced the creation
of an interim unity government that included members of both the previously
legal opposition party and previously outlawed political parties. This government
was highly contested. Reports of looting and violence continued, and the army
was stationed in the capital to maintain security. At the same time, Tunisians celebrated their newfound, and what they hope will be sustainable, freedoms. The
"Jasmine revolution," as it was quickly dubbed in the international press, was the
first of its kind in the Middle East North Africa (MENA) region.

As of late January 2011, the situation in Tunisia remains unstable and the future uncertain. Travelers to Tunisia and to other countries in the region, should
seek out the most recent information before traveling.

LAURA J. HAAS

NANCY B. MOCK

THOMAS EISELE

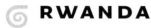 RWANDA

You cannot begin to appreciate Rwanda without first understanding the tremendous progress that has been made since the 1994 genocide — 100 days in which nearly a million Tutsi and moderate Hutu men, women, and children were massacred by an organized effort of the Hutu ruling party. Rwanda is currently on track to achieve all of its health-related UN Millennium Development Goals (MDGs) of reducing child mortality, improving maternal health, and successfully combating HIV, malaria, and other infectious diseases.[1] Much of Rwanda's success can be attributed to its impressive leadership and its results-based philosophy that emphasizes accountability and achievement. Many visitors to Rwanda, including those from its neighboring countries, are amazed by the progress Rwanda has made in the years following the genocide.

Brief Country History

A brief review of Rwanda's early development and the effects of colonialism will partially explain events leading up to the genocide. Rwanda was a highly centralized kingdom presided over by Tutsi kings. The relationship between the ordinary Bahutu, (also referred to as Hutu) Batutsi (or Tutsi), and Batwa (or Twa) people was one of mutual benefit derived mainly through the exchange of labor.[2] In 1899, Rwanda became a German colony; during World War 1, Belgian troops occupied the country, and in 1919, after the German defeat, the country was administered by the Belgians as a League of Nations mandate.[3] Rwanda was made a United Nations trust territory, administered by Belgium, in 1946. Under the Belgian colonial administration, a discriminatory national identification system based on ethnicity was introduced. Although originally favoring the minority Tutsi ruling elite, the Belgians quickly changed alliances as pressure for independence began, and supported a Hutu leading party, Parti du Mouvement de l'Emancipation Hutu (Party of the Hutu Emancipation Movement). Rwanda was granted political independence from Belgium's trusteeship on 1 July 1962. From 1959 onward, Tutsi were periodically threatened by massacres, resulting in numerous waves of outmigration throughout the following decades and increasing loss of life and livelihood based on ethnic divisionism.[4]

In the months leading up to April 1994, Rwandan media increasingly identified Tutsi as threats to Rwandan society, and ultimately called for their extermination. Upon the downing of President Habyarimana's plane on 6 April 1994, the extermination plan was set in motion, and roadblocks were instituted across the country. Ten Belgian soldiers serving in the UN Assistance Mission for Rwanda[5] were murdered immediately, initiating Belgium's withdrawal of its troops.[6] The remaining United Nations troops in the country, numbering less than 500 and led by Lieutenant General Roméo Dallaire, were unable to stop the massacre. Rwandan radio and newspapers daily reported names and license plates of Tutsi and moderate Hutu — those to be stopped and ultimately killed. In July 1994, the capital city of Kigali fell to the forces of the Rwandese Patriotic Army, the armed wing of the Rwanda Patriotic Front, led by Paul Kagame. Over three million refugees (accounting for roughly 40 percent of the population) fled to Tanzania and the Democratic Republic of the Congo. The Rwanda Patriotic Front established a government of national unity with four other political parties, followed weeks later by the formation of the Transitional National Assembly, which lasted until 2003, when a Parliament was formed.[7]

Rwanda is currently governed by a Parliamentary, multiparty system headed by President Paul Kagame, who was democratically elected in 2003 to a seven-year term. Rwanda's constitution was approved in 2003. The cabinet is comprised of twenty ministers representing all seven political parties. As of the September 2008 elections, women fill 55 percent of parliamentary seats. In fact, Rwanda's constitution mandates a minimum of 30 percent female representation in Parliament, the only country in the world to promote gender equity to this extent. Each minister is responsible for overall development for at least one of the thirty districts comprising Rwanda's four provinces (North, South, East, and West) and Kigali, the capital city. Rwanda is governed in a performance-based fashion where results are reviewed annually at a ministerial retreat, headed by President Kagame. Informed leadership has been critical to Rwanda's success.

Rwanda's visionary leadership plays a strong role in the country's progress, from its strong commitment to achieving the Millennium Development Goals (MDGs; see the glossary), to assuming ownership of its development process.[8] In the health arena, the Ministry of Health (MOH) provides strong direction and active coordination of donors and implementing agencies alike, ensuring that externally funded activities are in alignment with national health priorities. With Rwanda's emphasis on results, information and communication technologies are given high priority as tools to hasten development and provide timely information for planning and programming. Efforts are currently under way to expand connectivity throughout the country with the laying of fiber optic cable and to enhance bandwidth with the linking of the submarine cable out of Dar es Salaam, Tanzania, and Mombasa, Kenya.[9]

The Rwandan Context

Rwanda is the most densely populated country on the African continent. Roughly the size of Maryland, with only 26,338 square kilometers (10,169 square miles), it has a population of 10.746 million,[10] or 408 people per square kilometer (1056 people per square mile). The fertility rate is high, at 4.99 percent,[11] and the population has been increasing at an annual rate of about 2.7 percent. The population is expected to reach twelve million by the year 2012. Family planning is one of the government's top priorities. Over 80 percent of the population lives in rural areas, where there is a high level of poverty.[12] The age distribution is similar to that of many developing countries: approximately 42 percent of the population is under fifteen.[13] Hutus comprise the majority of the population (84 percent), followed by Tutsis (15 percent), and a small population of Twa, from the Pygmy group (1 percent).[14] However, in post-genocide Rwanda no official reference is made to ethnicity, a direct response to the divisionism so strongly linked to events leading up to the genocide. Currently, great efforts are made to ensure that genocide ideology is not taught in Rwanda's school system.

The civil war of 1994 caused a tremendous upheaval among the population, as the rebel Rwanda Patriotic Front made territorial gains from the north. Fearing reprisal, Hutus made a mass exodus from Rwanda, seeking refuge in Tanzania and the Democratic Republic of the Congo. Refugees found themselves in camps infiltrated and often controlled by the *Interahamwe*. In the local Kinyarwanda language, *Interahamwe* means "those who attack together," referring to the militant groups of the ruling party trained to carry out the genocide.[15] Although the fleeing refugees were invited back to Rwanda by the Rwanda Patriotic Front and promised security, many have not returned to their former villages but instead remain in refugee camps or have been absorbed into eastern part of the Congo. However, insecurity and instability remain constant elements of life in eastern Congo, especially along the northern border with Rwanda, as evidenced by recent flare-ups among rebel groups and government troops of the Congo.

As a response to these severe migrational shifts, Rwanda instituted a new structure to better manage and monitor the flow of its returning population. The local government registered all returnees, and any movement of the returnees required notification of local authorities. With the provision of housing support and availability of social services, returnees were encouraged to reestablish their homes in small clusters of ten or so, to complete a "block." Each block was supervised by a block captain. Ten or more blocks constituted a village, and clusters of five or more villages constituted a cell. An appointed local official endowed with the responsibility of monitoring population movement oversaw each level of organization. These small clusters of homes, which currently dot Rwanda's landscape, are a dramatic departure from the traditional style of village life. The new structure encourages larger, shared plots of land for cultivation; a sharp contrast to the more traditional organization of Rwandan villages, where a single home was surrounded by the family's fields and buffered from its neighbors.

Another important migration in Rwanda's recent, post-genocide history is the return of its diaspora. Throughout the decades since 1959, many of Rwanda's Tutsi took refuge all over the world—in Africa, Europe, and North America—to escape persecution at home, receiving training and education at the highest levels. Many of these highly skilled individuals have answered President Kagame's call to return to Rwanda and now lead its recovery and pursue its development goals by heading ministries, leading universities, and managing critical organizations in both the public and private sectors. The return of Rwanda's diaspora has had a tremendous impact on Rwanda's achievements in its post-genocide period, providing Rwanda a dynamic leadership not found elsewhere on the continent.

Economy, Income, and Education

Since 1994, Rwanda has maintained overall microeconomic stability and successfully implemented extensive reforms, including the establishment of independent regulatory agencies, stronger public expenditure management systems with independent audit agencies, and a strong commitment to anticorruption measures.[16] The government has embraced an expansionary fiscal policy to reduce poverty by improving health and education, encouraging foreign and domestic investment, and pursuing market-oriented reforms. As a result of these reforms, Rwanda's gross domestic product (GDP; see the glossary) has grown by 5 percent to 6 percent each year from 2002 to 2006, exceeded 6 percent in 2007, and was estimated to have grown 4.5% in 2009.[17] GDP per capita is estimated at $1,000 for 2008.[18] Still, energy shortages, instability in neighboring states, and lack of adequate transportation linkages to other countries continue to handicap economic growth.

Most Rwandans rely on subsistence agriculture. Agriculture provides jobs to 90 percent of the population and accounts for just over 40 percent of GDP.[19] Agricultural production remains low, with coffee and tea serving as Rwanda's primary foreign exchange earners. The country is investing heavily in its information and communication technology infrastructure and looking to tourism, especially mountain gorilla trekking, to enhance and diversify its economy. The contribution of the private sector to the economy and poverty alleviation remains limited. There are only about 400 private enterprises in Rwanda, of which half have fewer than fifty employees.[20] Rwanda is making good progress with its $9.7 billion economy.[21] The country has joined the Common Market for Eastern and Southern Africa, which seeks to promote regional trade and investment, and on 1 July 2007 formally joined the East African Community. Despite recent growth, Rwanda continues to be highly dependent on foreign aid to finance its development; external assistance has funded 60 percent of total public expenditures on average over the last three years.[22] The outlook for the Rwandan economy greatly depends on regional peace and stability and the success of the country's economic reforms.

The government of Rwanda devotes close to 20 percent of its annual budget to education.[23] The adult literacy rate (those age fifteen and above) is estimated at 70.4 percent of the population.[24] With the country's primary school net enrollment rate of nearly 96% in 2008, only four percent of children of primary school age were not attending school.[25] Non-fee barriers to primary education remain, including the cost of school uniforms and learning materials, which affect access to and retention in education.[26] Rwanda is actively striving to achieve the educational MDGs of attaining universal primary education by 2010, and education for all by 2015. In pursuit of these goals, the Ministry of Education (MOE) has implemented the following policies: fee-free education up to grade 9; prioritization of education for girls; teaching of HIV/AIDS education and life skills at all levels; and emphasis on science and technology, including that for information and communication.[27] In fact, Rwanda is one of the first countries to adopt a policy of one laptop per child and intends to distribute a laptop to half of its 2.5 million school children by 2012.[28]

Although originally a Francophone country, Rwanda has recently adopted English as the language for education and will no longer be using French in the classroom.[29] Beginning in early 2009, all educational institutions from primary to tertiary levels employed English in the classroom. Kinyarwanda, English, and French remain the official languages of Rwanda; Kiswahili is often widely used in commercial circles.[30]

The Healthcare System in Rwanda

The Rwandan healthcare system is based upon the foundations articulated by the Alma Ata Declaration of 1978. The Declaration recognizes health as an essential human right, and primary care as both a fundamental part of a country's health system and essential to the overall social and economic development of a country. Furthermore, recognizing that primary health care is usually the first contact a person has with the health system in any country, the Declaration suggests that the aim should be to bring care to the community level, as close as possible to where people live and work.[31] The mission of the MOH is to improve the health of Rwanda's population by strengthening the quality of services delivered and by providing access to treatment through universal health insurance coverage (discussed below).[32] Seven strategic areas are the country's focus for the health system through 2015:

Human resources development;
Availability of drugs, vaccines, and consumables;
Geographic accessibility of health services;
Financial accessibility of health services;
Quality of and demand for health services in the control of disease;
Strengthening national referral hospitals and treatment and
    research centers; and
Institutional capacity building.[33]

Health policy in Rwanda is guided first and foremost by the MDGS, with priority setting determined by Rwanda's government leaders and donor agencies. The MDGS are incorporated into the quantitative targets of Rwanda's Health Sector Strategic Plan.

In 2005, Rwanda undertook reforms that aligned the country's administrative and health districts, seeking to strengthen local-level capacities for planning, implementation, and monitoring, while reinforcing demand-driven service delivery. This restructuring created the following administrative levels: province (4), district (30), sector (416), cell (2,148), and village (14,975).[34] The health system is comprised of three levels: central, district, and sector. The central level is responsible for setting policy and providing support to the lower levels, especially with regard to program monitoring and reporting. Rwanda's recently revised national Health Sector Policy identifies the district as the basic operational unit of the health system.[35] The district level encompasses a district health team as well as a district hospital. The district health team is responsible for shaping district health plans and ensuring their implementation at the sector level. The sector is managed by the health center, which in turn oversees community health volunteers via cell level committees that are directed by a head of health and social affairs and one community health worker.

One of the greatest challenges facing Rwanda's health sector is the paucity of health manpower. Rwanda cites a health workforce density of 1.0 health worker/1000 population,[36] compared to 2.3/1000 for sub-Saharan Africa generally — well below the global norm of 2.5/1000 population recommended by the World Health Organization (WHO; see the glossary).[37] In 2007, Rwanda's doctor-to-population ratio surpassed 1 to 33,000 (up from 1 to 42,000 in 2005), and the nurse-to-population ratio rose to 1 to 1,700 (versus 1 to 3,138 in 2006).[38] These numbers do not include the large numbers of traditional healers who are a significant source of healthcare in Rwanda. Ensuring that manpower resources are of sufficient quantity and quality, and distributed according to the population's need, continues to pose real challenges.

Between 2003 and 2008, Rwanda will have trained an additional 1,790 healthcare professionals, including 327 doctors, 473 nurses, and 460 counselors.[39] However, distribution of the health workforce remains problematic, especially among doctors. As is often the case, more highly trained health providers prefer employment in urban areas as opposed to rural areas, which is where the large majority of the Rwandan population resides and the need is greatest. In response to this problem, authorities introduced a contract for medical students just beginning their residency program that obligates them to work for the MOH in a district hospital for two years; otherwise they will be required to reimburse the MOH for all expenses incurred during residency.[40] Rwanda possesses one medical school that currently enrolls 650 undergraduates, 90 postgraduates pursuing the master of medicine degree (specialty training), and 12 Ph.D. candidates. In 2007, for example, eighty-eight of the approximately 100 graduating medical students signed contracts before beginning their residency programs.[41]

The MOH has responded proactively to address inequities in access and quality of health services and to increase the accessibility of healthcare through community venues. For instance, the National Community Health Policy, which envisions Rwanda's health manpower needs and programs to 2020, increases the availability of primary health services at the community level through a nationwide network of health workers as the first line of primary care.[42] The plan is to equip each village with five community health workers (CHWS) comprised of the following: two general health workers known as *binomes*—one male and one female—one maternal health attendant, and two palliative care workers.[43] This large cadre of health workers will eventually mean 60,000 CHWS throughout the country.[44]

The country's recent success in providing treatment for malaria at the community level using CHWS opens potential new opportunities for expanding HIV treatment and care to rural areas using the CHW model. To improve access to care for the poor, the country has implemented free antiretroviral therapy (ART; see the glossary) and tuberculosis treatment, and introduction of user fees based on ability to pay.

The MOH is also committed to addressing financial accessibility issues through innovative mechanisms. An insurance plan, the Mutual Health Insurance Policy, is designed to increase financial accessibility to health services through community-level insurance plans.[45] In fact, Rwanda has experienced an impressive increase in access to and use of health services due, in part, to its health insurance program, called *mutuelles de Santé*. The program was initiated in 2003, in the provinces of Butare and Cyangugu, with an annual subscription rate of only 7 percent. It has since expanded to all areas of the country with a current estimated subscription rate of 92 percent.[46] Subscribers pay an annual fee or premium (currently $2 a year) for a basic package of services provided by the health center. This group health insurance plan is organized around bôth communities and professional networks. For example, the faculty of the National University of Rwanda and the Rwandan military have formed their own *mutuelles* to provide health insurance to their members. The improved utilization of health services is credited to mass population enrollment in the *mutuelle* program, mobility of care for those insured, improvements in healthcare providers' salaries, and the scale-up of performance-based financing in the country. In 2001, the rate of health service utilization was 24.7 percent; by 2007, four years after the implementation of the health insurance program, the rate of service utilization had increased to 71.9 percent, and is expected to increase as larger proportions of the population enroll in health insurance.[47] In spite of these successes, challenges remain to the *mutuelle* program: coverage of *indigents*, or the poorest of the poor, and ensuring that social insurance premiums actually cover the costs incurred by health facilities. In 2007, the MOH paid *mutuelle* subscription fees for 770,809 *indigents*. Many nongovernmental organizations (NGOS; see the glossary) working in the country, including numerous faith-based organizations (FBOS; see the glossary), also assume the subscription fees for those who cannot pay. Anecdotal evidence suggests that the insurance often does not adequately cover health costs; many health centers report high levels of consumption or repeat visits among insurance holders, often outpacing the premium's coverage of actual costs.

However, it is hoped that combining contributions from other Rwandan health insurance schemes such as those from the civil service and the military will improve program coverage and risk sharing.[48]

The MOH has implemented a contractual approach to results-based service delivery, referred to as performance-based financing (PBF). Results from piloting PBF in the districts of Butare, Cyangugu, and rural Kigali in 2001 indicated that the contractual approach of linking financial incentives for health workers to performance resulted in improved health outcomes.[49] Community PBF was initiated in all thirty health districts in December 2005, using the following six performance indicators:

1 Increased enrollment in the community health insurance program;
2 Reduction of maternal mortality;
3 Reduction of mortality due to malaria via increased utilization of treated bed nets;
4 Reduction of under-five mortality due to dehydration via increased utilization of oral rehydration solution;
5 Improvement of personal hygiene; and
6 Improved referrals on the part of CHWs.[50]

The challenges to community-level PBF include verification of the quantity and quality of CHW services delivered. Cooperatives for CHWs are being organized to serve as the contracting agency for organizing CHW data collection and reporting.

Leading Health Issues in Rwanda

Some promising initiatives in Rwanda demonstrate effective points of entry for healthcare in the community, such as home-based management of malaria, HIV/AIDS, TB, and nutrition; and community-based integrated management of childhood illnesses (or IMCI; see the glossary); and community distribution of family planning methods, all of which will be discussed in more detail below. The government's very proactive information and communication technology strategies promise to provide cell phone access to villages throughout the country.

Despite significant health funding going into Rwanda, health indicators are improving more slowly than the government anticipated. New health policies and decentralization of resources and healthcare delivery have not yet yielded health benefits to the degree desired. For instance, a 2007 survey of 538 public, government-assisted, and private facilities suggests the following major issues: poor infection control, lack of client counseling, and essential drugs frequently out of stock[51]—indicating the quality of care in Rwandan health facilities needs improvement. Some specific findings:

Only one-third of facilities have running water;

Only 22 percent of facilities, including 64 percent of hospitals, have soap;

In 3,000 consultations, 45 percent of providers did not warn clients that sexually transmitted infections increase risks of contracting and transmitting HIV infection;

In only 43 percent of consultations did providers discuss a pregnant woman's delivery plans, in spite of a major government initiative to encourage facility-based deliveries;

Over 40 percent of facilities offering diagnosis and treatment of malaria were out of stock of first-line antimalarials at some point in the six months before the survey; and

Almost three-fourths of facilities that treat HIV-positive individuals were out of stock of first-line antiretrovirals.[52]

Malaria

Malaria is the leading cause of morbidity and mortality in Rwanda, responsible for up to 50 percent of outpatient visits to the health system,[53] 43 percent of all episodes of illness, 43 percent of all deaths,[54] and nearly one-third of all deaths in children.[55] Nearly all infections are caused by *Plasmodium falciparum*, the most lethal form of the parasite (see malaria in the glossary).[56] Malaria also represents a significant health risk among women in their first and second pregnancies in Rwanda, especially in areas of stable transmission.[57] In 2005, there were 1.5 million uncomplicated malaria episodes reported through the public sector health system, although this likely represents an underestimate due to the low level of access and utilization of healthcare in the country at the time. By 2008, the intensive efforts undertaken to combat malaria, which are described below, have resulted in a marked decline in episodes of malaria to about 800,000 each year, and a 60% reduction in malaria deaths.[58]

Resistance to chloroquine and sulphadoxine-pyrimethamine has been widespread in Rwanda since the late 1990s.[59] In 2006, Rwanda switched its first-line drug for uncomplicated malaria to Coartem (artemether-lumefantrine).[60] The recommended treatment for severe malaria is currently intravenous quinine followed by oral Coartem. Community-based efforts to treat malaria in children ages six months to five years have demonstrated success in providing treatment within twenty-four hours of the onset of fever.[61]

Health centers in Rwanda have recently begun using rapid diagnostic tests for malaria to ensure infections are accurately detected and treated. The Rwanda National Malaria Control Program (the acronym is PNILP in French) has made the following interventions a priority for combating malaria across the country: indoor residual spraying; long-lasting, insecticide-treated bed nets; and prompt and effective case management using rapid diagnostic tests and Coartem. There has been a concerted effort to scale up these interventions in the past five years with assistance from the Global Fund to Fight AIDS, Tuberculosis and Malaria (see the glossary), the President's Malaria Initiative (see the glossary), the Belgian Technical Cooperation, the German Development Bank, and the Swiss Cooperation. The PNILP's four year national strategic plan for malaria has the following goals:

At least 80 percent of children under five and pregnant women sleep under an insecticide-treated bed net;

At least 80 percent of children under five with malaria receive affordable and effective malaria treatment within twenty-four hours of the onset of symptoms;

At least 90 percent of malaria cases attending health facilities receive case management according to national policy (a rapid diagnostic test and Coartem); and

At least 90 percent of malaria epidemics are identified and controlled within two weeks of the outbreak.

HIV/AIDS

Although malaria is by far the greatest burden of disease in Rwanda, HIV/AIDS receives far more attention and funding. After malaria, AIDS, pneumonia, and diarrhea are the next leading causes of morbidity and mortality among children under five. In fiscal years 2007 and 2008,

Rwanda received over $100 million annually from the President's Emergency Plan for AIDS Relief (PEPFAR; see the glossary) alone to support comprehensive HIV/AIDS prevention, treatment, and care programs.[62] Rwanda has demonstrated remarkable success in achieving its targets for addressing HIV/AIDS—and it has done this despite having endured the destruction of its health system during the 1994 genocide and possessing the highest burden of orphans and vulnerable children in Africa[63] (see the sidebar on the 1994 genocide and its aftermath for orphans and vulnerable children).

The HIV prevalence rate among adults (ages fifteen to forty-nine) in Rwanda is estimated at 2.8 percent,[64] with rates slightly higher in urban areas and among women. For example, the 8.6 percent HIV prevalence rate among women in Kigali is most likely due to a post-genocidal legacy of gender-based violence.[65] Rwanda has aggressively expanded HIV services and integrated them with other key health services in the country, including reproductive health and family planning. Currently, over 60,000 HIV-positive individuals are treated with ART through a network of 171 ART sites.[66] By 2007, a total of 285 health facilities were providing prevention of mother-to-child transmission services, and 313 were providing voluntary counseling and testing.[67] Ninety-five percent of pregnant women attending antenatal care were tested in 2007; approximately 106,000 women are tested each year.[68] Care and support services are provided through an extensive network of associations of people living with HIV who conduct home visits and provide referrals to healthcare facilities.

HIV/AIDS is a national priority for the Rwandan government, as it recognizes the impact of this disease on the country's prospects for growth and development. The government has developed a national HIV/AIDS action framework in collaboration with its major partners in the fight against AIDS—the Global Fund to Fight AIDS, Tuberculosis and Malaria; the Joint United Nations Programme on HIV/AIDS (UNAIDS; see the glossary); the U.S. government via PEPFAR; WHO; and the World Bank—to ensure a shared vision and coordination of effort and resources. Rwanda's National Policy on HIV and AIDS has created an environment with a coherent, systematic, and efficient national response to HIV/AIDS.[69]

THE 1994 GENOCIDE AND THE
CHALLENGES FACING RWANDA'S
ORPHANS AND VULNERABLE CHILDREN
AND YOUTH

INNOCENT TUMAINE KAYITARE

Rwanda was a calm, simple African nation, largely rural, with its massive population barely surviving on a stingy economy based on tea and coffee. That was until the year 1994, when the hateful acts of a few brought a dark cloud onto Rwanda. Now and forever, Rwanda shall be linked with the term "genocide." During Rwanda's 100 days of horrific genocide, many Rwandans lost their parents: either one or both parents were killed, leaving the young ones with no one to take care of them. Some children were raped and sexually abused, a leading cause of HIV/AIDS among orphans and other vulnerable youth in Rwanda. Many children lost parents to internal displacement in Rwanda and its neighboring countries, and others to imprisonment. These factors have all contributed to the development of households headed by children and youth in Rwanda.

In Rwanda, a vulnerable child is defined as a person under eighteen, exposed to conditions that do not permit her or him to fulfill his or her fundamental rights for harmonious development. An orphan is defined as a child who has lost one or both parents. Rwanda has struggled with the long-term consequences of the genocide. Poverty is pervasive: 51 percent of the population lives below the national poverty line. Children are among the most severely affected, with orphaned and abandoned children being particularly vulnerable. Orphans constitute approximately 29 percent of all children under eighteen in Rwanda. Nearly 40,000 children are the heads of their households, and over 90,000 children live in child-headed households. HIV/AIDS has greatly worsened these problems, with an estimated 20 percent of all orphans having lost parents to the disease.[70] The effects of these factors on young people and on the society are numerous: economic stagnation or decline as children grow into unskilled workers; morbidity and malnutrition because children's basic needs are not met; and increased spread of HIV as young people concentrate on survival rather than protection.[71]

Children living in youth-headed households are less likely to attend school and constitute the largest proportion of the estimated 104,000 (10 percent) children who are out of school in Rwanda. Girls suffer the most: significant numbers of orphaned girls never start or complete school, in spite of Rwanda's fee-free education policy.[72]

Children living in youth-headed households are more vulnerable to physical and mental health problems and behavioral problems (due to a lack of appropriate adult guidance and comfort), and often show developmental delays. Without a caring adult to advocate for their interests, they are also more vulnerable to physical and sexual abuse, property and land grabbing, and labor exploitation.[73]

Responsibility for orphans in Rwanda customarily falls to the patrilineal side of the family, but other types of care arrangements are possible and close friends can be considered part of the family. Rwandans suggest the 1994 genocide eroded these traditional care structures.[74] The social disruption of the genocide is unmistakable. In roughly 100 days, nearly a million people were massacred, often at the hands of their neighbors, friends, and even family members. Death, imprisonment, exodus, and repatriation of Rwandans (many of whom had been in exile long before the genocide) shattered communities. These events strained social networks and community solidarity, posing serious challenges to the care of orphaned youth. Stigmatization is also a great challenge to community care for orphans. Children may be stigmatized due to circumstances surrounding parental death or absence and HIV/AIDS, or even as victims of genocide; these children lack care and sometimes are considered outcasts from society.

The growing numbers of vulnerable children pose a problem to the traditional ways of incorporating these children into extended family structures. Children who are marginalized from community supports and protective family care systems have decreased capacity to function in society. Lacking traditional coping systems, supports, and other services, vulnerable children are exposed to rights abuses. These abuses take a number of forms, including sexual abuse, exploitation, and harmful labor; children are often deprived of fundamental rights with regard to their protection and their development.[75]

The government of Rwanda has adopted numerous strategies to address and raise awareness of the problems of orphans and other vulnerable children and youth, and to change the perception from "their problem" to "our problem." Legislative procedures and regulations have been instituted to assure consistent child-rights-focused programs and services in favor of orphans and other vulnerable children. Innovative community mentor systems have been established throughout the country to provide adult support and interaction for child-headed households.[76]

INNOCENT TUMAINE KAYITARE is a program assistant for Tulane University's Rwanda Country Office. He provides technical assistance to the National Malaria Control Program (PNILP) and coordinating assistance to the Tulane School of Social Work and National University of Rwanda joint activities in social work. He is a graduate of Makerere University in Uganda with a BA in Sociology and a minor in Social Administration. His professional interests include disease monitoring and evaluation, especially HIV/AIDS and malaria, and social work approaches to understanding and finding solutions to problems affecting Rwandans.

Tuberculosis

In 2008, 7227 new cases of TB were identified among Rwandans, an increase of roughly 1.5 percent over a three-year period.[77] The increase in TB in Rwanda is driven by the HIV epidemic. However, as TB and HIV activities are increasingly integrated at the health facility level, co-infection rates are more quickly identified. In 2008, 96 percent of TB patients were tested for HIV, and 34 percent were identified as co-infected.[78] Currently, fifty-two health facilities are involved in the follow-up of multidrug-resistant tuberculosis (MDR TB; see the glossary) patients on ambulatory treatment. Typically MDR TB treatment lasts eighteen to twenty-four months. The treatment success rate for the cohort of fifty MDR TB patients that started treatment in 2006 reached 86 percent, demonstrating Rwanda's successful follow-up of these patients.[79] In 2008, eighty-one patients started second-line treatment for MDR TB during the course of the year.[80]

Rwanda's TB case detection rate in 2007 was considered low (48 percent compared to the WHO target of 70 percent);[81] however, the treatment success rate in 2008 (86 percent) surpassed the 85 percent target.[82] Case detection and treatment success rates require improvement if the spread of TB is to be halted and reversed.[83] At present, TB surveillance and testing is conducted in all thirty districts and by the four reference hospitals, as well as by a small number of private services.[84]

By 2008, coverage of 70 percent of health districts and employing CHWS to deliver community-based DOTS, the WHO-endorsed approach to TB control, (see the glossary) to TB patients benefited 72 percent of the population.[85] In addition to their curative role, DOTS CHWS detect persons with chronic cough for referral to the heath center and raise awareness about TB in the local communities.[86]

Family Planning and Reproductive Health

Maternal and infant mortality remain important health priorities in the country. Rwanda's high infant mortality rate (81.6 infant deaths per 1,000 live births), coupled with high fertility, low rates of contraceptive use (17 percent among married women), and high maternal mortality (1,300 maternal deaths per 100,000 live births) are all areas of concern receiving attention by the government. The government is dedicated to several strategies to reduce maternal mortality, including: improving access to and utilization of family planning services to help birth spacing and reduce unintended pregnancy; encouraging pregnant women to give birth in a health facility; and using trained CHWS to identify and refer potentially high-risk deliveries to a health facility. Efforts to increase deliveries in health facilities are showing success; the rate of assisted deliveries increased to 55 percent in 2007 (up from 49 percent in 2006). The percentage of pregnant women who attended antenatal care increased to 94 percent in 2007 (from 82 percent in 2006); more than 75 percent of pregnant women complete at least one prenatal visit at a health facility.

Beginning in 2009, the MOH implemented an innovative approach to determining the reasons behind continued maternal deaths and understanding how such deaths can be prevented — a sort of "social autopsy," examining community, social, and health service factors contributing to each maternal death.[87] In addition to health agents and local authorities, neighbors and other community members are questioned about the circumstances leading up to a maternal death so as to help avoid future occurrences.

Family planning is a priority area of health intervention. The MOH has developed a National Program for Reproductive Health, a national strategy for implementation of interventions for family planning and reproductive health, and established a technical working group on family planning comprised of national and international partners. The MOH strives to integrate family planning into other healthcare services, most notably HIV/AIDS, and specifically into ART and contraceptives. Modern contraceptive methods are available in all health facilities.

Malnutrition

With increasing population pressures, high levels of poverty, and food insecurity in many of the rural areas throughout the country, the nutritional situation remains alarming in Rwanda. Although severe malnutrition decreased slightly, from 24 percent in 2000 to 22 percent in 2005, chronic malnutrition increased from 42 percent to 45 percent during the same period.[88] According to Rwanda's 2005 Demographic and Health Survey, chronic malnutrition affects 45 percent of children under five. A national policy on nutrition has been adopted, and information, education, and communication activities on the benefits of fruit and vegetable gardens for individual households were carried out in 2007.[89] Other activities to combat malnutrition include:

Two campaigns annually to distribute vitamin A, insecticide-treated bed nets, and deworming medications;
Establishment of a food security surveillance system;
Promotion of exclusive breast-feeding;
Promotion of small-animal husbandry, including chicken raising in all rural households;
Promotion of better food preparation practices, using locally available foods.[90]

Community Integrated Management of Childhood Illnesses

In response to its elevated infant and child mortality rates, Rwanda has embraced the Integrated Management of Childhood Illnesses (IMCI; see the glossary) as a key strategy to combating childhood death and disease. To be truly effective in reducing child mortality, IMCI must move beyond the health facility level and provide case management of illness at the community level, while also focusing on prevention and reduction of undernutrition.[91] The CHW is identified as the key agent in carrying out this strategy. The country's plan for IMCI envisions a network of trained CHWs with at least one CHW per ten households, each of whom will coordinate with a multidisciplinary committee linked to the health center.[92] CHW responsibilities will focus initially on: delivery of curative care; case management of fever and diarrhea; distribution of insecticide-treated nets, vitamins, and oral rehydration solution; and education of families on basic wellness practices.[93] Rwanda's initial success with IMCI is evidenced by clear reductions in infant and child mortality, although rates still remain unacceptably high.

Key Agencies, Partnerships, and Coordination in Rwanda

The Rwandan health sector is characterized by high-level, active involvement of the government and extensive donor support, much of the latter provided via vertical projects to specific disease interventions. There can be significant variation in funding to different diseases; for instance, $47.8 million annual funding for HIV/AIDS compared to $780,000 for TB.[94] In 2004, growing dissatisfaction with the project approach led the government of Rwanda to improve coordination of external assistance through the development of the Sector Wide Approach across sectors.[95] The approach is a partnership between the Rwandan MOH and its development partners to ensure that external assistance is in alignment with Rwanda's long-term vision for health sector development.

Under a memorandum of understanding, the government of Rwanda and its development partners come together in pursuit of national priorities via the Health Sector Cluster Group, which is co-chaired by the MOH as the government representative and the Belgian Technical Cooperation as the lead donor. Cluster members include one representative from each of the bilateral and multilateral development partner agencies, the lead national and international health NGOS, the national religious community active in the health sector, as well as representatives from the HIV/AIDS Cluster Group, Ministry of Finance and Economic Planning, and the Global Fund to Fight AIDS, Tuberculosis and Malaria's country coordinating mechanism.[96] Thus, the government of Rwanda and its development partners come together to ensure

Rwanda's ownership of its development process, to encourage transparency between partners, and to improve efficiency and effectiveness of resource allocation in the health sector.

Tulane University Partnerships in Rwanda

Tulane University has been a health development partner with Rwanda since 2000, actively working in the higher education, policy, and service delivery components of Rwanda's health system. Tulane cofounded the National University of Rwanda's School of Public Health in 2001 and continues to develop the school's institutional capacity. This ongoing partnership focuses on: advocacy for policy reform; strategic planning, administrative and management systems development; educational and training programs; and faculty development. Joint educational and training programs include: an executive M.P.H. program for in-service training of health professionals; a sandwich program for doctoral studies, allowing students to conduct their thesis research in several short periods within the country; and an innovative program to provide recent university graduates with the opportunity to gain important workplace experience through the Rwanda HIV/AIDS Public Interest Fellowship program (see the sidebar on workforce development).

Tulane University has a significant, ongoing role in a broad range of health sector projects in the country. For instance, Tulane leads the Child Survival, Malaria, and Nutrition component of the Twubakane Decentralization and Health Project, begun in 2005; provides critical technical assistance for the rollout of clinical and community integrated management of childhood illnesses; and collaborates with Rwanda's National Malaria Control and Prevention Program (PNILP) to strengthen sentinel surveillance systems and epidemic detection and response systems, train district malaria control and prevention officers, conduct the 2009 Malaria Indicator Survey, and provide doctoral training of PNILP center level staff at Tulane University.

Conclusion

What you notice when first arriving at Kigali International Airport in Rwanda is the absolute lack of chaos as you maneuver through immigration, baggage claim, customs, and transport options. The calm and orderliness of the airport is a reflection of what you will find through-

INNOVATION IN
WORKFORCE DEVELOPMENT
The Rwanda HIV/AIDS Public Interest Fellowship

MAGGIE BAINGANA KALININGONDO
AND CHANTAL I. MURENZI

In Rwanda, the problem of trained human resources is more complex than in any other African country due to the lingering demographic impact of the genocide, combined with the devastating human toll HIV/AIDS is taking on the population. Today, Rwanda suffers from an inadequate critical mass of trained people in many areas. HIV/AIDS has traditionally been regarded primarily as a medical and epidemiological issue restricted to the health sector, but it needs to be addressed as a societal issue, with attention to the underlying socioeconomic dynamics and sociocultural problems. Guided by this vision, and motivated by the urgent need to fill the gap in trained human resources, and in order to provide opportunities for practical experience for graduating students, the Rwanda HIV/AIDS Public Interest Fellowship program was started.

The program prepares young professionals from a variety of disciplines with the skills and experiences to serve as competent managers of HIV/AIDS programs in Rwanda. To do this, the program draws recent university graduates from non-health backgrounds and places them in a paid two-year internship with an MOH agency or NGO working in HIV/AIDS. Fellows are trained in HIV/AIDS, leadership, and project management. The program is highly competitive: fifteen fellows are selected from over 400 applications annually, and over fifty host agencies apply each year for one of the fifteen fellows. The program provides practical training at six-month intervals, delivered by the National University of Rwanda School of Public Health, to develop the fellows' knowledge and skills in leadership and management of HIV/AIDS programs, and in computing, so as to strengthen workplace efficiency and fill a capacity gap among host agencies.

Among the three fellowship cohorts (forty fellows) to date, most are retained by their host agency, becoming midlevel managers in the not-for-profit sector. Some go on to pursue graduate studies, and a few hold senior leadership positions (for instance, country coordinator of the Network of Religious Confessions in the Fight against HIV/AIDS, and country director of Orphans of Rwanda, an international NGO).

Due to the program's success, it has been replicated in the public and private sectors in Kigali. The Ministry of Public Service and Labor started a youth employment program using the fellowship as a model two years ago. In late 2008, Tulane was asked to expand this model of institutional capacity development to a broader spectrum of institutions in Rwanda's health sciences sector, specifically those responsible for health workforce development in medical education, social work, and nursing.

MAGGIE BAINGANA KALININGONDO, LLB, LLM, serves as Tulane's Technical/Legal Advisor for the Rwanda HIV/AIDS Public Interest Fellowship Program, and provides assistance to the Ministry of Health's TRACnet technical team in the drafting of training modules and other documents for the national HIV/AIDS monitoring system. She joined Tulane University/Rwanda Country Office in 2004, after working for four years with the Attorney General of Rwanda on the prosecution of genocide cases and other war crimes. Ms. Kaliningondo holds a Master of Laws degree (LLM) in Government Law and Public Policy from the University of the Pacific, California, and a Bachelor of Laws degree (LLB) from Makerere University, Uganda.

CHANTAL I. MURENZI, B.SC. is Technical Assistant for Tulane's Rwanda Country Office, where she has provided technical support to the implementation of the Rwanda HIV/AIDS Public Interest Fellowship Program (RHPIFP) since 2007. Mrs. Murenzi holds a degree of Bachelor of Science in Chemistry from Clark Atlanta University and a Diploma in Pharmacy from Université Libre de Bruxelles (Independent University of Brussels), Belgium.

out the rest of the country. Courteous baggage carriers will either assist you for a flat rate or provide you with your own luggage trolley. Taxi drivers quietly wait in their coats and ties to drive you into town — there is no need to haggle over prices, and in fact, very little bartering takes place in Rwanda, even at the lively but orderly markets. On the short ride into town, you will be struck by the cleanliness of the streets, swept practically daily, and the wide, cobblestone sidewalks. There are no plastic bags becoming one with the earth as you often find in Africa; plastic bags have been outlawed in Rwanda for a number of years now, and the results are obvious. (If your duty free purchases are in plastic bags, you'll need to leave the plastic behind before leaving the airport.)

There is a certain quietness about Kigali after hours, even on Friday and Saturday nights. There are few people on the streets late at night, but it is still quite safe to walk around, even for visitors. Security on Rwandan streets is a priority for the government, and the highly visible police are there to facilitate. There is zero tolerance for corruption, and traffic stops are just that: checks for documentation and basic functioning of your vehicle—windshield wipers, indicators, do you have all you need to change a flat tire, including your emergency triangle? In many ways, Rwanda is a very easy place to work—well organized, with easy and inexpensive communication via cellphones and Internet. It welcomes visitors, especially those who are willing to work hard toward Rwanda's development.

Rwanda is a beautiful and fertile country, known as "the land of a thousand hills." The country has six volcanoes, twenty-three lakes, and numerous rivers, some flowing into the great Nile,[97] and three national parks with a diversity of flora and fauna. The Volcanoes National Park is home to the endangered mountain gorilla and the late Dian Fossey's Karisoke Research Center. Visitors can trek through the mountains, accompanied by trained guides, to spend an hour with gorillas, in very close proximity. Akagera National Park, a game reserve in the low savanna along the border with Tanzania, provides wildlife including giraffes, water buffalo, hippos, and zebras. Nyungwe National Park, located in the southwest region of Rwanda, encompasses the largest island of montane forest remaining in East and Central Africa, an ancient center of unparalleled biodiversity with more than 100 species of orchid and numerous primates.[98]

COUNTRY DATA : RWANDA

Millennium Development Goal indicators are italicized.

TABLE 6.1 : **POPULATION AND HUMAN DEVELOPMENT**

POPULATION	
Total	10.746 million
Population growth rate	2.78%
Net migration rate/1,000 population	2.17
Urban	18%
Rural	82%
AGE STRUCTURE	
0–14 years	42.1%
15–64 years	55.4%
65+ years	2.4%
Median age (years)	18.7
MAJOR ETHNIC GROUPS	
Hutu	84%
Tutsi	15%
Twa	1%
RELIGIONS	
Christian	93.6%
Muslim	4.6%
Indigenous/traditional	3.1%
Other	1.7%
HUMAN DEVELOPMENT	
Human Development Index	0.435
Human Development rank[a]	165th
Freedom House Index	Not free
Political Rights score[b]	6
Civil Liberties score[b]	5
Human Poverty Index	36.5%
Human Poverty rank[c]	161st

Notes: [a] out of 179 countries; [b] 1 = most free, 7 = least free; [c] out of 177 countries.

TABLE 6.2 : **GOVERNMENT AND ECONOMY**

GOVERNMENT

Independence	1 Jul. 1962 from Belgian-administered UN trusteeship
Type of government	Republic
Voting rights	Age 18, universal

CAPITAL — Kigali

CURRENCY — Rwanda franc (RWF)

ECONOMY

Gross Domestic Product (GDP) (in PPP US $)	9.706 billion
Annual GDP growth	4.5%
GDP per capita (in US $)	$1,000
Gini Index	46.8
Population living below PPP $1/day	60.3%
External debt service as % of GDP	1.1
Public debt as % of GDP	17.4
Official development assistance (ODA) per capita (in US $)	$63.7
Foreign direct investment as % of GDP	0.4

LABOR FORCE

In agriculture	90%
In industry and services, combined	10%
Unemployment rate	NA

TABLE 6.3 : **GEOGRAPHY AND ENVIRONMENT**

LAND COMPOSITION

Land area	26,338 sq. km. (10,169 sq. mi.)
Size comparison	Slightly smaller than Maryland
Terrain	Grassland and hills; mountainous with declining altitude west to east, landlocked
Ecological hazards	Periodic droughts, volcanic mountains in northwest

LAND USE AND RESOURCES

Permanent crop land	45.6%
Arable land	10.2%
Agricultural products	Coffee, tea, pyrethrum (insecticide), bananas, beans, sorghum, potatoes, livestock
Natural resources	Gold, tin ore, tungsten, methane, hydropower
ENVIRONMENTAL ISSUES	Deforestation from uncontrolled cutting of trees for fuel, overgrazing, soil exhaustion and erosion, poaching

INFRASTRUCTURE

Population with access to improved water source	35%
Population using improved sanitation	42%
Roadways unpaved	81.0%

TABLE 6.4 : **HEALTH**

LIFE, BIRTH, AND DEATH

Life expectancy at birth (male/female)	49.2/51.8
Birth rate/1,000 population	39.67
Death rate/1,000 population	14.02
Infant mortality rate/1,000 live births	*81.61*

PERSONNEL AND INFRASTRUCTURE

Physicians/100,000 population	3.03
Hospital beds/10,000 population	16

HEALTH ECONOMICS

Total expenditure on health per capita (PPP US $)	$126
Public expenditure on health as % of GDP	4.3%

DISEASES

Most common vector-borne diseases	Malaria
Most common food- and water-borne diseases	Bacterial diarrhea, hepatitis A, typhoid fever
TB incidence/100,000 population	*397*
TB prevalence/100,000 population	*562*
New TB cases HIV-positive	37%
New TB cases multidrug-resistant (MDR)	3.9%
1-year-olds fully immunized against TB	89%
Estimated malaria cases annually	800,000
Malaria death rate/100,000 population	NA
HIV prevalence rate in adults	*2.8%*
AIDS deaths in adults annually	*7,800*
People living with HIV	150,000
AIDS orphans	220,000

MATERNAL HEALTH

Fertility rate (children born per woman)	5.25
Contraceptive prevalence rate (married women 15–49)	*17.4%*
Maternal mortality rate/100,000 births	*1,300*
Lifetime risk of maternal death, 1 in:	*16*
Births attended by skilled birth attendant	*39%*

CHILD HEALTH

Mortality rate of children < 5/1,000 live births	*160*
1-year-olds immunized against measles	*95%*
Children < 5 using insecticide-treated bed nets	*5%*
Children < 5 with fever treated with antimalarial drugs	*3%*
Newborns protected against tetanus	82%

Children < 5 underweight for age	*23%*
Children < 5 under height for age	*48%*
Population undernourished	*33%*

TABLE 6.5 : LANGUAGE, EDUCATION, AND LITERACY

LANGUAGES

Kinyarwanda	Official language (universal Bantu vernacular)
French	Official language
English	Official language; language in the classroom
Kiswahili	Spoken in commercial centers

LITERACY

Adult literacy rate (population age 15+ who can read and write)	70.4%

EXPENDITURE

Public expenditure on education as % of GDP	3.8

EDUCATION

Net enrollment in primary education[d]	*95.9%*
School life expectancy, in years (male/female)[e]	9/8

[d]Net enrollment rate in primary education is measured as the number of children of official primary school age who are enrolled in primary education as a percentage of children in the official primary school age population.

[e]School life expectancy is the total number of years of school (from primary through tertiary education) that a child can expect to receive.

Principal Sources for Data in Appendix Tables 6.1–6.5

Central Intelligence Agency, *The World Factbook* (https://www.cia.gov/library/publications/the-world-factbook/).

UN Millennium Development Goals Indicators Database (http://millenniumindicators.un.org/unsd/mdg/).

UNDP Human Development Report, 2007/2008 (http://hdr.undp.org/en/reports/global/hdr2007-2008/).

UNICEF. The State of the World's Children 2009 (http://www.unicef.org/publications/index_47127.html)

NOTES

1. United Nations, "MDG Monitor: Rwanda" (http://www.mdgmonitor.org/country_progress.cfm?c=RWA&cd=646).

2. Official Website of the Republic of Rwanda, History (http://www.gov.rw/page.php?id_rubrique=9).

3. Ibid.

4. Ibid.

5. United Nations Assistance Mission for Rwanda was an effort by the United Nations to aid the implementation of the Arusha Accords, (signed August 4, 1993), aimed at ending fighting between Tutsis and Hutus in the country. The mission placed several hundred UN military forces in Rwanda from October 1993 to March 1996.

6. Roméo Dallaire, with Brent Beardsley, *Shake Hands with the Devil: The Failure of Humanity in Rwanda* (New York: Carroll and Graf, 2003).

7. Government of Rwanda. History of People.

8. Paul Kagame, "Remarks by His Excellency, Paul Kagame, President of the Republic of Rwanda," Address to the Development Partners Meeting, Hotel Intercontinental, Kigali, Rwanda, 22 November 2006.

9. Murenzi, Romain. Presentation at the US — Africa Initiative for Higher Education. Delivered at the Serena Hotel, Kigali, Rwanda, October 2008.

10. Central Intelligence Agency. The World Factbook. Rwanda (https://www.cia.gov/library/publications/the-world-factbook/geos/rw.html).

11. Central Intelligence Agency, World Factbook, Rwanda.

12. Ibid.

13. Ibid.

14. Ibid.

15. Dallaire, *Shake Hands with the Devil*, 531.

16. The World Bank, Country Data Report for Rwanda 1996–2008. (info.worldbank.org/governance/wgi/pdf/c188.pdf).

17. Central Intelligence Agency, The World Factbook, Rwanda.

18. Ibid.

19. Ibid.

20. The World Bank, Country Data Report for Rwanda.

21. Ibid.

22. Ibid.

23. UNESCO Institute for Statistics, "UIS Statistics in Brief: Education in Rwanda" (http://stats.uis.unesco.org/unesco/TableViewer/document.aspx?reportId=121&IF_Language=eng&BR_Country=6460).

24. Central Intelligence Agency, The World Factbook, Rwanda.

25. United Nations Statistics Division, Millennium Development Goals Indicators Database, "Net enrollment ratio in primary education, 2008" (http://data .un.org/Data.aspx?d=MDG&f=seriesRowID%3A589).

26. Ministry of Education, Republic of Rwanda, "Fee-free Education" (http:// www.mineduc.gov.rw/spip.php?article21).

27. Ministry of Education, Republic of Rwanda, "The Strategic Plan of the Ministry of Education" (http://www.mineduc.gov.rw/spip.php?article20).

28. Ministry of Education, Republic of Rwanda, "Can One laptop per Child Transform Rwanda's Economy?" (6 July 2010; http://www.mineduc.gov.rw/spip .php?article79).

29. Felly Kimenyi, "Kagame Reiterates Need to Use English as Education Medium," *New Times*, Kigali, Rwanda, (15 October 2008; http://allafrica.com/ stories/200810150230.html).

30. Central Intelligence Agency, The World Factbook, Rwanda.

31. Declaration of Alma Ata, International Conference on Primary Health Care, Alma-Ata, USSR, (6–12 September 1978; www.who.int/hpr/NPH/docs/ declaration_almaata.pdf).

32. Ministry of Health, Republic of Rwanda, (http://www.moh.gov.rw/).

33. Ibid.

34. Catherine Fort, "Decentralization and Local-level Governance in Health: Some Experiences from Rwanda and the Philippines," paper presented at the USAID Health Systems 20/20 Health Governance Workshop, Washington, D.C., 13 June 2007.

35. Government of Rwanda, "Health Sector Policy" February 2005 (http:// www.eac.int/health/index.php?option=com_docman&task=doc_details&gid= 2&itemid=47).

36. Government of Rwanda, "Human Resources for Health Strategic Plan 2006–2010" (http://www.hrhresourcecenter.org/node/1610).

37. World Health Organization, "The World Health Report 2006. Working Together for Health" (http://www.who.int/whr/2006/en/index.html).

38. World Health Organization, "WHO Country Collaboration Strategy Rwanda, 2009–2013," Brazzaville, Republic of the Congo: WHO Regional Office for Africa, 2009 (http://www.afro.who.int/en/rwanda/who-country-office -rwanda.html).

39. Republic of Rwanda," HIV/AIDS Treatment and Care Plan, 2003–2007" (13 June 2003; http://www.hrhresourcecenter.org/node/204).

40. World Health Organization, "WHO Country Collaboration Strategy Rwanda, 2009–2013."

41. Ibid.

42. Republic of Rwanda, Ministry of Health, "National Community Health

Policy," 2008 (http://www.google.com/search?ie=UTF-8&oe=UTF-8&sourceid=
navclient&gfns=1&q=http%3B%2F%2F+www.usaid.gov%2Frw%2Four_work
%2Ffor...%2Fnationalcommunityhealthpolicy.pdf).

43. Ibid.

44. Ibid.

45. Republic of Rwanda, Ministry of Health, "Mutual Health Insurance Policy
in Rwanda," December 2004.

46. Donald G. McNeil, Jr., "A Poor Nation, With A Health Plan," The New
York Times, 14 June 2010 (http://www.nytimes.com/2010/06/15/health/
policy/15rwanda.html).

47. Republic of Rwanda, Ministry of Health, "Annual Report 2007." Kigali,
Rwanda, April 2008.

48. D. E. Logie, M. Rowson, and Felix Ndagije, "Innovations in Rwanda's
Health System: Looking to the Future," Lancet, 372 (2008): 256-61.

49. R. Soeters, L. Musango, and B. Meesen, "Comparison of Two Output Based
Schemes in Butare and Cyangugu Provinces with Two Controlled Provinces
in Rwanda," Butare, Rwanda and Antwerp and The Hague, The Netherlands,
Global Partnership on Output-Based Aid (GPOBA) The World Bank and Rwanda
Ministry of Health, 6 August 2005 (http://www.multicountrypbfnetwork.org/
Comparison.pdf).

50. Republic of Rwanda, Ministry of Health, "Community Performance Based
Financing: User Guide," 2008 (http://www.pbfrwanda.org.rw/index.php?option
=com_docman&task=search_result&itemid=29).

51. Republic of Rwanda, Ministry of Health and the National Institute of Statistics (in collaboration with USAID and Macro International), "Rwanda Service
Provision Assessment (RSPA), 2007," 18 November 2008 (http://statistics.gov
.rw/index.php?option=com_content&task=view&id=205&itemid=202).

52. Ibid.

53. U.S. Centers for Disease Control and Prevention and USAID, "President's
Malaria Initiative: Malaria Operational Plan (MOP): Rwanda FY 2007" (Kigali:
CDC and USAID, 2008).

54. J. P. Van Geertruyden, et al., "Malaria Infection among Pregnant Women
Attending Antenatal Clinics in Six Rwandan Districts," Tropical Medicine &
International Health 10, no. 7 (2005): 681-88.

55. U.S. Centers for Disease Control and Prevention and USAID, "President's
Malaria Initiative."

56. M. E. Loevinsohn, "Climatic Warming and Increased Malaria Incidence in
Rwanda," Lancet 343, no. 8899 (1994): 714.

57. Clinical observations of large numbers of pregnant women in malaria
endemic areas have shown that a pregnant woman's susceptibility to clinical

malaria decreases with parity. That is, during a first pregnancy and sometimes a second a woman has an increased risk of severe infection. The risk appears to diminish with each successive pregnancy. The exact reasons for this are not well understood, although it is suspected that women lack immunity to a specific pathogen to which they are exposed during pregnancy, and acquire immunity over sequential pregnancies (http://www.scielosp.org/pdf/bwho/v8on5/a14v8on5.pdf); A. Hammerich, et al., "Unstable Malaria Transmission and Maternal Mortality Experiences from Rwanda," *Tropical Medicine & International Health* 7, no. 7 (2002): 573–76; Van Geertruyden et al., "Malaria Infection among Pregnant Women Attending Antenatal Clinics in Six Rwandan Districts." *Tropical Medicine & International Health* 7, no. 7 (2002): 681–688.

58. Rwanda: Winning the Fight against Malaria, "The Rwanda Success Story" (http://www.malariafreefuture.org/rwanda/success.php).

59. Hammerich et al., "Unstable Malaria Transmission and Maternal Mortality Experiences from Rwanda."

60. U.S. Centers for Disease Control and Prevention and USAID, "President's Malaria Initiative."

61. Pascal Musoni, "Community Based Malaria Treatment in Rwanda," paper presented at the Thirty-fourth International Global Health Conference, Washington, D.C., 31 May 2007.

62. U.S. President's Emergency Plan for AIDS Relief, "Partnership to Fight HIV/AIDS in Rwanda" (http://www.pepfar.gov/countries/rwanda/index.htm).

63. U.S. President's Emergency Plan for AIDS Relief, "FY2008 Country Profile: Rwanda" (http://www.pepfar.gov/press/countries/profiles/116316.htm).

64. UNAIDS, "Report on the Global AIDS Epidemic" (2008). (http://www.unaids.org/en/KnowedgeCenter/HIVData/GlobalReport/2008/default.asp).

65. United Nations Development Programme, "Turning Vision 2020 into Reality: From Recovery to Sustainable Human Development; National Human Development Report, Rwanda 2007" (http://www.rema.gov.rw/soe/chap1.php).

66. Rwanda, Ministry of Health, "Rapport Annuel, 2007."

67. Ibid.

68. Ibid.

69. Rwanda, Office of the President, National AIDS Control Commission, "National Policy on HIV and AIDS, Final Draft." 5 November 2007. (http://www.aidsportal.org/Article_details.aspx?ID=6246).

70. B. E. Antoine, and D. Pinault, "Nkundabana: A Model for Community-based Care for Orphans and Vulnerable Children by Care International in Rwanda," paper presented at the Sixteenth International AIDS Conference, Toronto, 13–18 August 2006.

71. Ibid.

72. V. Taton, et al., "Investing in Rwanda: Effective Choices for Orphans and Girls in Primary Education" (UNICEF, Division of Policy and Planning, May 2007; http://www.unicef.org/socialpolicy/index_45565.html).

73. L. Brown et al., "Psychosocial Benefits of a Mentoring Program for Youth Headed Households in Rwanda," (Population Council, 2007; http://www .popcouncil.org/countries/rwanda.asp).

74. Renee Thurman et al., "Barriers to the Community Support to Orphans and Vulnerable Youth in Rwanda," *Social Science & Medicine* 66, no. 7 (2008): 1557–67.

75. Rwanda, Ministry of Local Government, Information and Social Affairs, "National Policy for Orphans and Other Vulnerable Children."

76. Ibid.

77. Rwanda, Ministry of Health, "Rapport d'activités de l'année 2008" (February 2009).

78. Ibid.

79. Ibid.

80. Ibid.

81. Rwanda Economic Development and Poverty Reduction Strategy (EDPRS). Health Sector Working Group. "EDPRS Self Evaluation Report: Health, Population, and HIV/AIDS," 17 May 2006.

82. Rwanda, Ministry of Health. TRAC Plus. TB Unit. Op.cit.

83. Ibid.

84. Rwanda, Ministry of Health "Rapport Annuel, 2007."

85. Rwanda MOH. TRAC Plus, TB Unit. Op.cit.

86. Ibid.

87. Interview with Richard Sezibera, the Rwandan minister of health, 14 February 2009.

88. Rwanda, Ministry of Health, "Rapport Annuel, 2007."

89. Ibid.

90. Ibid.

91. World Health Organization, Integrated Management of Childhood Illness. "Multi-Country Evaluation: Main Findings" (http://www.who.int/imci-mce/ findings.htm).

92. Rwanda, Ministry of Health, "Plan stratégique de la prise en charge integrée des maladies de l'enfance (PCIME) " (2006).

93. Ibid.

94. Rwanda, Ministry of Health, "Donor Mapping Study: Preliminary Results" (2005).

95. Rwanda, Ministry of Health. "Rapport Annuel. 2007."

96. Rwanda Economic Development and Poverty Reduction Strategy (EDPRS). Health Working Group. Op.cit.

97. Government of Rwanda (GOR). Official Website of the Republic of Rwanda — Tourism. (http://www.gov.rw/.)

98. Ibid.

SUGGESTED READING OR VIEWING

Briggs, Philip. *Rwanda: The Bradt Travel Guide*. 3rd ed. Guilford, Conn.: Bradt Travel Guides, 2006.

Courtemanche, Gil. *A Sunday at the Pool in Kigali*. Translated by Patricia Claxton. Edinburgh: Canongate, 2003.

Dallaire, Roméo, with Brent Beardsley. *Shake Hands with the Devil: The Failure of Humanity in Rwanda*. New York: Carroll and Graf, 2003.

Gourevitch, Philip. *We Wish to Inform You That Tomorrow We Will Be Killed with Our Families: Stories from Rwanda*. New York: Farrar, Straus and Giroux, 1998.

Kinzer, Stephen. *One Thousand Hills: Rwanda's Rebirth and the Man Who Dreamed It*. Hoboken, N.j.: Wiley, 2008.

Peck, Raoul, dir. *Sometimes in April*. DVD. HBO Home Video. 10 May 2005. (http://www.hbo.com/).

President's Emergency Plan for AIDS Relief (PEPFAR). "2008 Country Profile: Rwanda." http://www.pepfar.gov/press/countries/profiles/116316.htm.

Raymont, Peter, dir. *Shake Hands with the Devil: The Journey of Roméo Dallaire*. DVD. 1 February 2005. Montreal, Canada, The National Film Board of Canada.

Republic of Rwanda, Ministry of Health. Publications. http://www.moh.gov.rw/index.php?option=com_docman&itemid=14. (Includes national policy documents, laws, annual reports, national health accounts, 2005 Demographic and Health Survey, and more.)

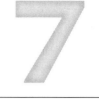

MICHELLE SCOTT

PALAV BABARIA

NEEL R. GANDHI

 # SOUTH AFRICA

South Africa is a country of diversity and contrasts. Not only is its population racially diverse, but it encompasses a wealth of varying cultures, from French villages in the Western Cape,[1] to the Minstrel Carnival in Cape Town, and to Zulu homesteads in KwaZulu-Natal. Economic diversity ranges from upper-class wealth comparable to that in the United States or Europe, to abject poverty similar to some of the poorest countries in Africa and the world. South Africa is best known for its modern political history — in particular, the brutal segregation of the apartheid regime, followed by a peaceful democratic transition under the leadership of Nelson Mandela. The legacy of South Africa's political history continues to influence all aspects of modern-day life. In this chapter we will try to paint a picture of today's South Africa, along with a historical context in which to understand it.

Our vantage point into this fascinating country is from the small rural hamlet of Tugela Ferry, in the province of KwaZulu-Natal. KwaZulu-Natal is best known in South Africa for its beautiful beaches on the Indian Ocean, which straddle Durban, the busiest port city in Africa. Unfortunately, KwaZulu-Natal is also home to the country's worst epidemics of HIV, tuberculosis (TB), and drug-resistant TB. These contrasts, pervasive throughout modern South Africa, can be tangibly experienced in the 180-kilometer (112-mile) journey from Durban to Tugela Ferry.

Durban is a beautiful tropical city with a diverse population of whites, Indians, and blacks, and all of the comforts of an American or European city — modern beachside hotels and resorts, shopping malls, and cafes. The drive north of Durban passes through the Natal Midlands — a landscape of scenic rolling hills, dotted with lush sugarcane and timber farms. These estates, once havens for British colonists escaping the humid Durban summers, are now emblematic of South Africa's continued economic strength (South Africa remains the world's fifth largest producer of sugar). After passing Greytown, a small town that serves as a commercial crossroad for this agricultural region, there is a bend in the road where Natal turns into KwaZulu, the relocated heartland of the Zulu people.

As you cross over a hill, a nearly distinct line separates the green of Natal from the red, rocky, desert land of KwaZulu. This region is home to descendants of the great Zulu tribe who were devastated by wars with white settlers in the nineteenth century, and oppressed by homeland policies of the apartheid regime in the twentieth century. Now the region is among the poorest and least developed districts in South Africa, with unemployment rates as high as 40 percent. Most inhabitants live in traditional homes of packed mud and thatched roofing, the majority lacking running water or electricity. The HIV epidemic has ravaged this region; HIV prevalence rates among pregnant women reach 30 percent, and nearly every family has lost someone to AIDS. The recent discovery of a drug-resistant TB epidemic in this region only adds to the suffering and the challenges of improving healthcare for this highly underserved population.

Just as the journey from Durban to Tugela Ferry that we've described embodies South Africa's sociopolitical history through its changing landscape, the historical, political, and socioeconomic factors we describe in this chapter have shaped the current status of health in South Africa. Our viewpoints are inevitably shaped by our experiences as American clinicians and researchers working at a district hospital in a small rural town. Yet Tugela Ferry epitomizes the post-apartheid challenges that characterize much of South Africa and have played a key role in fueling the HIV/AIDS and TB epidemics in this country. To understand the challenges, you need to start by understanding the history.

A Short History of Early South Africa

Indigenous San and Khoikhoi nomadic tribes resided in South Africa for thousands of years. In the fourth century, they were joined by

Bantu-speaking agrarian tribes that migrated south from Central Africa. These groups remained largely undisturbed until 1497, when the Portuguese explorer Vasco de Gama established the spice route around the Cape of Good Hope. The Portuguese left the area unsettled. However, the Dutch East India Company began to use the coast of southern Africa as a rest stop along its trade routes. A formal Dutch colony was established in 1652, which eventually came to be known as Cape Town. The Dutch imported thousands of slaves from India, Madagascar, and Malaysia to use as indentured labor on the vast plantations they developed. Descendants from these slaves comprise the Indian populations in KwaZulu-Natal and Cape Malay in modern-day Cape Town.

Expanding their empire on the African continent in the late eighteenth century, the British conquered Cape Town and quickly enforced British policies over the local populations. Conflicts erupted between the newly arrived British colonists and the earlier Boer settlers. The Boers (Dutch for farmers)—a conglomeration of Dutch, German, French, and Flemish colonists, many of whom had fled religious persecution in Europe—had settled in the Cape Town area as farmers during Dutch rule and become a distinct cultural group. Their descendants are now called Afrikaners. British-imposed Anglican laws and restrictions on slave ownership did not sit well with the Calvinist Boer farmers. In an effort to escape both British rule and increasing conflicts with the local indigenous Xhosa tribe, the Boers migrated northward on the "Great Trek" in the 1830s and 1840s, eventually founding the Orange Free State and Transvaal.

The migration of European colonists beyond the Cape colony led to violent battles between the British and the Boers and between white settlers and the native Xhosa and Zulu tribes, as white settlers infringed on traditional tribal lands. The Boer discovery of diamonds near Kimberley in 1867, and gold in 1884, resulted in the first (1880) and second (1899) Anglo-Boer wars, fought over control of the mines. A compromise was reached in 1902, consolidating all the disparate Boer and British outposts and leading to the formation of the Union of South Africa in 1910. Under British rule, the union formalized the century-long racial discrimination between whites and blacks with the ratification of the 1913 Natives' Land Act. This law, limiting black ownership of land to a small percentage of the country and preventing new land acquisition by blacks, was the beginning of the country's race-based policies.

The Apartheid Era

Apartheid by Law

The Afrikaner National Party came to power in 1948, on a platform of racial segregation or *apartheid* (separateness, in Afrikaans). In 1950, the party classified and segregated all individuals on the basis of race: black, white, Indian, Asian, and Coloured, referring to individuals of mixed descent. Under the Group Areas Act, families were forcibly re-located from long-established communities to newly created segregated townships outside of the cities. Black, Coloured, and Indian communities that occupied prime coastal property were issued eviction notices; these areas were razed and converted into whites-only neighborhoods. Once vibrant, multicultural, and multireligious communities, such as Cape Town's District Six, were disassembled and destroyed.

After a whites-only referendum in 1961, South Africa left the British Commonwealth and became the Republic of South Africa. As other African countries were breaking from colonial rule and the continent swelled with the pride of African nationalism, the South African government tightened its grip on freedoms for people of color, fearing that in the hands of black leaders the country would follow the path of many newly independent African nations and embrace socialist or communist ideals.[2] Over nearly forty years, the apartheid government systematically segregated all communities and created racial hierarchies. Under this hierarchical system, Indian, Asian, and Coloured populations were generally afforded greater access to jobs, education, and other resources than black South Africans.

Under the Bantu laws of the 1950s to 1960s, black South Africans were denied education, jobs, quality medical care, and land. With the Pass Law Act of 1952, blacks were forced to carry identification passes at all times; these passes determined where a given individual was allowed to live, work, and socialize (even drink beer). Black South Africans were restricted in movement and limited in education to keep them a subservient class and prevent uprisings against the apartheid system.

In 1970, black South Africans were deemed no longer to be citizens of the Republic of South Africa. They were transported to the "homelands" —areas of rural land intended to serve as independent black nations (similar to Native American reservations in the United

States). These areas were severely lacking in municipal infrastructure, sanitation, electricity, and arable land.

Political Resistance

As the Afrikaner National Party increased the stringency of its race-based policies, the African National Congress (ANC) began to organize the growing anger, frustration, and resentment of black South Africans. Created in 1912, the ANC was created as a nontribal political group to unify all black communities for black South African rights. The ANC led a civil disobedience "defiance campaign" in 1952, inspired by the non-violent efforts of Mahatma Gandhi in India. Participants purposefully violated segregationist laws; over 8,000 people were arrested, including Nelson Mandela. New laws passed by the Afrikaner National Party in 1953 prohibited such protests.

However, the ANC remained firmly dedicated to a vision of a multi-cultural South Africa. In 1955, a group of black, Indian, and white ANC members wrote the Freedom Charter, declaring that "South Africa belongs to all who live in it, black and white."[3] The Africanist faction of the ANC, believing that South Africa was a country for blacks, split from the ANC in 1959, forming the Pan-Africanist Congress (PAC). Both PAC and the ANC continued to lead mass protests against apartheid, often resulting in police shootings of unarmed protestors, as happened in Sharpesville in 1960 when over sixty protestors were shot dead by police. In 1964, Nelson Mandela, along with several other prominent ANC leaders, was arrested and convicted on charges of sabotage and sentenced to life in prison on Robben Island.

The 1970s saw a resurgence of protest, as student leaders such as Steve Biko championed the black consciousness movement. In 1976, the township of Soweto became the site of an organized strike boycotting the requirement for black schools to use only Afrikaans as the language of instruction. The shooting death of a thirteen-year-old student by armed guards led to riots that lasted weeks and resulted in the deaths of 600 people and injuries to 4,000. The protests were brutally repressed, and the government declared further restrictions on black South Africans.

South Africa came under harsh international criticism for its racist policies in the 1960s and 1970s. The country was banned from the Olympic Games in 1964, a ban that lasted until 1992 — following the repeal of the country's apartheid laws the previous year. While the country faced sanctions and divestment from the external international community, protests and demonstrations escalated internally.

Facing widespread international and domestic pressure, the Afrikaner National Party responded in 1990, by removing the ban on the ANC and releasing Nelson Mandela from prison. F. W. de Klerk, the final president of the apartheid government, worked with Mandela to end apartheid and institute a more democratic government. In 1994, black South Africans were able to vote for the first time; the ANC won a landslide election, electing Nelson Mandela to the presidency.

Modern South Africa: The Rainbow Nation

South Africa's relatively recent and rapid transition to democracy was remarkable. So, too, was Nelson Mandela's smooth transition to power, marked by tolerance, forgiveness, and a focus on unity. In his inaugural address, Mandela stated: "We enter into a covenant that we shall build a society in which all South Africans, both black and white, will be able to walk tall, without any fear in their hearts, assured of their inalienable right to human dignity—a rainbow nation at peace with itself and the world."[4]

In his effort to create a raceless society in a country once identified by the strict division of white and black, Mandela's government faced enormous obstacles. Despite the largest gross domestic product (GDP; see the glossary) in Africa ($120 billion), South Africa had a large deficit and massive inequalities between the country's racial groups. Mandela tackled the challenge of reversing the discriminatory policies of the apartheid era, but it was his focus on forgiveness and unity that would be his legacy. He courted former apartheid leaders, spoke Afrikaans at public events, and firmly believed that the nation could not heal without addressing the grievances committed under the apartheid regime.

The South African Truth and Reconciliation Commission, established in 1995 by the government of national unity, aimed to help deal with the crimes of apartheid by investigating—not prosecuting—severe human rights violations committed between 1960 and 1994 by all perpetrators, including the apartheid regime, the ANC, and resistance movements. All individuals who came forward to confess their crimes were granted amnesty from prosecution.

The commission's 1998 report acknowledged apartheid as a crime against humanity, in line with United Nation's 1974 International Convention on the Suppression and Punishment of the Crime of Apartheid, and recognized that the country's new constitution formed a "bridge between the past of a deeply divided society characterised by strife, conflict, untold suffering and injustice and a future founded on the recognition of human rights, democracy and peaceful co-existence."[5] By giving testimony before the commission victims had an opportunity to seek resolution. While the process did not punish perpetrators, the commission is largely considered the vehicle by which South Africa has been able to unify and move past the events and discrimination of the apartheid era.

Following Mandela as president, Thabo Mbeki had a far more controversial presidency (1999–2008), marked by increasing racial tensions, allegations of government incompetence and corruption, and failures to address the AIDS epidemic (discussed later in this chapter). Not unlike the United States, race and socioeconomic disparities remain at the forefront of South African political discourse. Although workplaces, schools, and public spheres are now more integrated and a black middle class has steadily grown in size, racial and economic tensions remain. Recent political dialogue has begun to raise notions of reverse discrimination. Although whites make up only 9 percent of the nation's population, they represent 45 percent of its income. Eighty percent of new jobs are reserved for blacks, and with the advent of black affirmative action has come resentment from whites, Indians, and Coloureds at what they perceive as unfair discrimination. Many argue that rather than entering a raceless era, as promoted in the Freedom Charter, South Africa has simply reversed racial discrimination, with all opportunities and advancement reserved for blacks. The concerns were captured by Jody Kollapen, chair of South Africa's statutory Human Rights Commission: "Mandela was the kind of president who made white people feel more secure and comfortable because of his strong focus on reconciliation. The Mbeki presidency was characterized by a strong need to deliver and to transform, which was why we saw programs that pushed greater equity, and once you started talking greater equity, it meant making inroads into white people's interests."[6] In reality, even with affirmative action policies, the gap between blacks and whites in economics, education, and employment remains very large.

The Population and Current Socioeconomic Conditions

South Africa is one of the few nations in the world that is simultaneously first world and third world. Private hospitals in Durban provide state-of-the art healthcare, while rural children in Tugela Ferry die of kwashiorkor (a form of severe, protein-energy malnutrition). In this country, quality of life is strongly related to race and rural-urban geography.

South Africa's diverse population of 49 million is 79 percent black, nearly 10 percent white, 9 percent Coloured, and 2.5 percent Indian or Asian; it includes a sizable migrant population from other areas of the continent. The majority of the population is Christian, but many black South Africans still participate in traditional religious practices. KwaZulu-Natal, and particularly Durban, hosts the majority of South Africa's sizable Indian population, most of whom are Hindu or Muslim.

When the ANC first came to power in 1994, it established the Reconstruction and Development Program with the aim of achieving greater equality through job creation, redistribution of land, and the development of major housing and social services. Through the program, the government has built thousands of new homes to improve living conditions for the nation's poor. These basic but adequate structures have resulted in vast improvements, but large inequalities still exist: 41 percent of South Africans still have no access to improved sanitation, 18.5 percent have no electricity, and 29.1 percent still use paraffin or wood for cooking.[7] Sturdily constructed housing, reliable electricity, piped water inside dwellings, and flush toilets are most available in urban areas and among white populations; rural residents and black populations remain the most disadvantaged in terms of basic housing and utilities.

National adult literacy is estimated at 86.4 percent; however, functional literacy (defined as reading and writing on at least a seventh-grade level) is likely lower. Although 98 percent of all seven- to fifteen-year-olds attend school, only 24 percent of children complete twelfth grade. The most common reasons why children stop attending school are inability to pay school fees and the need to work to help support the family. Despite sliding scales for school fees, many families cannot afford even nominal fees, given the high rates of unemployment and rising food and living costs. Inequalities are apparent in schooling: 22 percent of black South Africans have no schooling, compared to 8.3 percent of Coloureds, 5.3 percent of Indians and Asians, and 1.4 percent of whites.

Unemployment is a significant issue. Various estimates are that from 22.9 percent to 40 percent of the population is unemployed, depending on the region of the country, with rates reaching as high as 75 percent in the former homelands and rural areas. Although the economy is growing and there is a great demand for labor, it is for labor at a skill level for which many black South Africans lack education or training, a reflection of the lasting damage inflicted by the Bantu laws, which limited education and training for the vast majority of black South Africans. With rates of unemployment in rural areas approaching or exceeding 70 percent, there is massive internal migration toward urban centers in search of employment. As the most prosperous nation on the continent, South Africa has long been a beacon for African immigrants fleeing poverty and political instability in their home countries. There are an estimated three million Zimbabweans and two million other African immigrants living in South Africa. Tensions have risen as the need for unskilled labor becomes scarce, and the growing number of immigrants creates even greater competition for jobs. These tensions culminated in anti-immigrant riots in May 2008. While the xenophobic riots are an extreme example of the effects of migration on communities, the more subtle impact of employment and migration patterns on individual and public health is illustrated in the case study of miners included in this chapter.

South Africa's Human Development Index (HDI; see the glossary) has decreased during the post-apartheid era (from 0.73 in 1995 to 0.68 in 2007), largely due to widening gaps between rich and poor, as well as the devastating impact of HIV/AIDS on life expectancy. While democracy has led to the creation of a black elite and a growing black middle class, the income gap between rich and poor has been steadily widening. Per capita income is $5,760; however, white households earn six times the income of black households. Forty-eight percent of South Africans now fall below the poverty line. While some South Africans are prospering, the poor are not only being left behind but are actually growing in number.

The Healthcare System in South Africa

As illustrated in the miners' case study, public health is often heavily influenced by economic, political, and historical factors. The juxtaposition

THE MINES : A CASE STUDY

Every December the population of rural towns such as Tugela Ferry doubles as the men return home for the holidays from Johannesburg, the mines, and other industries or job hunts. In this region, where more than 70 percent of households are run by women during the rest of the year the return of husbands, fathers, and sons is eagerly anticipated. But December is also fraught with the darker side of the migration for work. Hospital emergency rooms are flooded with the outcomes of alcohol-induced brawls, gunshots, and sexual assaults. The largely female population seen in the HIV clinics throughout the year is replaced with HIV and TB co-infected men, who have received little care during the year. It is difficult to manage these chronic diseases with only a yearly visit. These are the results of the complex interactions between South Africa's political history, current socioeconomic conditions, and migration linked to jobs.

South Africa's mining industry comprises almost 20 percent of its GDP: gold, diamonds, platinum, chromium, and coal are the natural resources of the country. South Africa is the world's second largest producer of gold and one of the largest producers of diamonds. Since the discovery of gold and diamond deposits near Kimbereley in the late 1800s, these natural resources have driven the political development of the country, served as a major source of wealth for early white settlers, and contributed significantly to the massive personal fortunes of individuals such as Cecil Rhodes. Under apartheid, rural black populations were utilized as cheap sources of labor for white-owned mines and factories. With limited education and employment options for black South Africans under apartheid, working in the mines was one of the few opportunities for supporting their families — a trend that continues today. Separated from their families, which eventually destroyed the social fabric of black South African communities, men were housed in single-sex dormitories and forced to work in what were considered some of the world's most dangerous mines. The large male workforce and single-sex housing invariably attracted prostitution to these areas; large percentages of miners had multiple sexual partners.

South Africa's mines, factories, and farms have attracted approximately 2.5 million migrants from within South Africa and bordering nations. More than 90 percent of these men still live in same-sex hostels surrounded by brothels and continue to work under substandard conditions in the mines. They are paid poorly and have inconsistent access to health care. What has changed in the post-apartheid era is the pattern of migration. During apartheid, migration was tightly regulated by the state. The abolition of these restrictions has allowed migrant men to return home more frequently, resulting in increased contact between migrant and rural hometown populations. There is significant migration for employment other than mining, as well. Durban, an urban center, has seven single-sex hostels that have a total of 43,000 beds. The impact of this migrational shift is that in rural areas of KwaZulu-Natal, the male and female populations are roughly equal at birth, but by age thirty-two women comprise from 65 percent to 70 percent of the region's population, depending on the community.

These migrational patterns and the working and social conditions of miners are responsible for a sizable percentage of HIV/AIDS transmission, an increase in sexually transmitted infections, and a rise in occupation-related exposures to TB and other pulmonary diseases. Migrant men are 2.4 times more likely than non-migrants to be HIV-infected; HIV-infected men are also more likely to live away from their wives and have multiple sexual partners than HIV-negative men.[8] By 1998, the prevalence of HIV was 20 percent in mine workers and 70 percent among prostitutes in areas surrounding the mines. By 2000, 90 percent of all miners were migrants who returned home to their families once a year for dedicated holidays. At the start of the HIV epidemic, transmission was largely unidirectional, from migrant men to their rural partners; currently, in 30 percent of discordant couples, the female is the HIV-infected partner.[9] This trend reflects the trajectory of the epidemic; migration patterns may have been responsible for the bulk of early transmission, while local transmission now fuels the incidence.

It is estimated that South Africa will lose one-third of its workforce by 2020 to HIV/AIDS, with the mining and extraction industries most severely affected. Earlier this decade, diamond and gold mining companies began to realize the economic impact of HIV/AIDS; lost productivity and sick days are estimated to be 10.7 percent of payrolls. Anglo Gold, one of the country's largest gold producers, initiated one of the country's first antiretroviral therapy (ART; see the glossary) programs for its workers in 2002, calculating that while ART is expensive, a workers' ART program would save the company money compared to the loss of workers.

Outside of the private sector, small projects have attempted to target health-related interventions to miners and prostitutes. However, a large-scale regional or national response will be necessary to make a significant impact on the HIV epidemic and on public health. In addition to education, condom distribution, and access to quality healthcare, societal changes such as the elimination of single-sex housing for migratory workers and rural economic development that reduces the need for migration for work are needed to impact the HIV epidemic.

of the first world and third world in South Africa is not limited to socioeconomics; it is also seen in the healthcare system. The world's first human heart transplant was performed in South Africa roughly forty years ago. Yet on a population level, basic measures of health such as infant mortality (44.4 infant deaths per 1,000 live births) continue to be among the worst worldwide. These contrasts are best understood in a political and historical context.

The Healthcare System in the Apartheid Era

Under the former apartheid government, access to healthcare and the quality of care received were racially, geographically, and economically prescribed. Formerly, the Department of National Health and Population Development was the principal government agency responsible for health and allocated money to three separate Ministries of Health Services and Welfare that served whites, Indians, and Coloureds, respectively, and to ten homeland departments responsible for healthcare within each racially black "Bantu state."[10]

Each ministry had its own provincial and programmatic administrative offices. Thus, within a given province there were three separate offices for whites, Indians, and Coloureds, in addition to bureaus for the homelands located within that province. The provincial office oversaw a variety of health programs such as TB control, child and maternal care, family planning, dental services, nutrition, and preventive care services. Using TB services as an example, each province had four separate TB program offices that did the same administrative work. In a given community, there were at least four separate TB clinics providing duplicate services, and each of these four clinics functioned independently of other programs that provided relevant services such as preventive care.

This public-sector system resulted in redundant programs, wasted resources, and uncoordinated care. Coexisting private health services added yet another dimension of complexity. Cedric de Beer, who has written extensively about healthcare in South Africa, assessed the system saying: "The health services are not, in the first instance, attempting to meet the needs of the people. Rather, their operations reflect the needs and policies of the Apartheid state."[11]

Not surprisingly, then, resources were unequally distributed by race, color, and geographic location. Although 44 percent of the population was black and lived within the ten homelands, the homelands received only 19 percent of the 1990-91 national health budget. Health expenditures were 11.5 times greater for whites than for blacks. Greater resources were allocated to urban areas, placing the rural homelands at a further disadvantage. In 1990, the doctor-to-population ratio was 1 to 700 people in urban areas, 1 to 1,900 in rural areas, and 1 to 10,000–30,0000 people in the homelands.

Most black South Africans needed access to basic primary, preventive, and community services—programs that received the least funding. For the rural black population, access to healthcare was difficult since most people either lived out of reach of a health center or had to travel long distances on foot to get to the nearest clinic, which was often understaffed and lacking basic resources such as refrigeration, medical supplies, communication, or transport in cases of emergency. The new healthcare system continues to grapple with the difficulty of providing adequate care to the rural poor.

The Current State of Healthcare

The democratic government elected in 1994 inherited a highly fragmented and unequal public healthcare system. Since 1994, South Africa's health policy has focused on reducing health inequities and delivering health services through comprehensive and integrated primary care services. A new national healthcare system was restructured and decentralized under the district health system model—a model endorsed by the World Health Organization (WHO; see the glossary) as best suited for delivering integrated primary healthcare. The model removed the responsibility of care from the provincial level and redirected it to individual health districts, which act semi-autonomously to deliver healthcare at the community level. This has resulted in 300 new clinics nationwide and a three-fold increase in per capita expenditure on primary healthcare (from $7.73 in 1992–93 to $24.40 by 2005-06).

Each health district contains local clinics, community health centers, and hospitals. A patient's first point of entry into the healthcare system is through the local clinic or community health center. A clinic is open eight hours a day and offers only primary healthcare. A community health center provides the same services as a clinic, in addition to having twenty-four-hour maternity and emergency services. In these two settings, patients are able to access a range of primary healthcare programs, including mother and infant care, immunizations, family planning, reproductive and sexual health services, and management of chronic illnesses. Clinics and community health centers are nurse-run, with weekly to monthly visits by a doctor deployed by the district. Patients with more complex problems are referred to the local district hospital for care. The goal of the restructured health system is to increase access to a comprehensive package of services considered by the government to be basic rights of its citizens.

Despite greater funding for primary healthcare, the current healthcare system is still plagued by an insufficient workforce and competing, parallel public and private systems. Compared to other middle-income countries, South Africa has a shortage of healthcare workers. In 2004, there were 8 physicians for every 10,000 people in South Africa, compared to 12 per 10,000 population in Brazil, 14 per 10,000 in Turkey, 25 per 10,000 in Poland, and 30 per 10,000 in Argentina. Restructuring has shifted the focus toward a nurse-based primary care system, since the country's nurse-to-population ratio of 41 per 10,000 people exceeds that of countries of similar incomes. However, the number of nurses is still insufficient to handle the massive patient load. In addition, the health workforce continues to be unequally distributed between urban and rural areas, and between the private and public sectors. Approximately 39 percent of the population lives in rural areas, which rely almost exclusively on public-sector care. The majority of healthcare professionals, however, are concentrated in urban areas, with nearly 66 percent of doctors in the private sector.

The Department of Health has tried various strategies to attract healthcare workers to the public sector and to rural sites, including a "scarce skills and rural" bonus for doctors willing to work in underserved and rural areas; a compulsory year of community service in underserved areas for physicians, pharmacists, and dentists; and recruitment of foreign doctors to work specifically in underserved areas. Regardless of the incentives provided, healthcare workers continue to be drawn to urban areas where they can more readily find housing and schools adequate to meet their families' needs. Those that do take jobs in rural areas usually do so only temporarily. Consequently, staff turnover is very high, and healthcare workers are often not invested in the communities they serve.

Emigration of health personnel, a common theme throughout the African continent, is also draining South Africa of health manpower. In 2001, approximately 8,921 South African doctors were working abroad in Australia, Canada, New Zealand, the United Kingdom, and the United States, while only 11,332 doctors were working in the public sector within South Africa. Many feel driven out of the country by work overload, high crime rates, and exposure to AIDS and other endemic infectious diseases.

Parallel Private and Public Health Systems

Privatization of healthcare in South Africa began in the 1970s and 1980s, and became official government policy in order to curb rising costs and encourage better utilization and coordination of healthcare. By the early 1990s, 28 percent of all hospital beds and 60 percent of doctors were in the private sector, providing care to the wealthy or medically insured who constituted less than 20 percent of the population. Today, the private system continues to consume disproportionate health resources at the expense of the majority of the population. While 15 percent of the population currently receives healthcare through the private sector, this sector receives 62 percent of the total healthcare expenditure. In addition, a significant portion of public funds is spent on training health professionals (through education subsidies and student scholarships) who go into the private healthcare sector after completing their training. It is common practice for doctors to run private practices on the side, while completing their commitments to the state.

Leading Health Issues in South Africa

It should be no surprise that South Africa has just as large a problem with diseases of poverty, such as TB and diarrheal diseases, as it does diseases of excess, such as diabetes and cardiovascular disease. While these illnesses touch all racial and ethnic groups, there is a distinct pattern: chronic diseases are more common in white and Indian populations, and infectious diseases and violence are more prevalent in black and Coloured communities. Each set of diseases is closely associated with the socioeconomic status of the population. The disturbing part of this dichotomy, however, is that the majority of medical resources are spent on diseases of excess, even though diseases of poverty affect the majority of the population. In this section, we provide a brief overview of the leading health issues (of both poverty and excess) in South Africa.

HIV/AIDS

South Africa is home to the largest number of HIV-infected people worldwide. Approximately 5.7 million South Africans are infected, and it is estimated that the national HIV prevalence is between 15.4 percent and 20.9 percent. Some regions of South Africa have antenatal HIV rates exceeding 40 percent. The South African government has been notoriously slow in addressing the HIV epidemic. As a result, the country has seen a rapid growth in disease prevalence. In fact, it was not until the ANC party faced a reelection campaign in 2003–4, and the possibility of poor polling as a result of their handling of the HIV epidemic, that they felt pressure to address it. The timeline and history of HIV/AIDS in South Africa, shown in the accompanying sidebar, dramatically illustrate the rapid growth of the epidemic in the face of the government's hesitancy to act.

The government's initial denial of HIV was met with outrage from both local and international communities. While a complacent response to the suffering of black South Africans would not have been unusual

1982: First recorded case of HIV in South Africa.

1985: South African government sets up the country's first AIDS Advisory Group in response to rising HIV prevalence.

1990: First national antenatal survey to test for HIV finds 0.8 percent of pregnant women are HIV-infected. An estimated 74,000 to 120,000 people in South Africa are living with HIV.

1991: The number of diagnosed heterosexually transmitted HIV infections equals the number transmitted through sex between men. Since this point, heterosexually acquired infections have dominated the epidemic.

1992: Nelson Mandela addresses the newly formed National AIDS Convention of South Africa, the government's first significant response to AIDS. The purpose of the convention is to develop a national strategy to cope with AIDS. The free National AIDS Helpline was founded.

1993: The national Department of Health reports that the number of recorded HIV infections had increased by 60 percent in the previous two years and is expected to double in 1993. HIV prevalence rate among pregnant women is 4.3 percent.

1995: International Conference for People Living with HIV and AIDS is held in South Africa. The South African Ministry of Health announces that some 850,000 people (2.1 percent of the total population) are believed to be HIV-infected.

1996: HIV prevalence rate among pregnant women is 12.2 percent.

1997: A national review of South Africa's response to AIDS epidemic finds a lack of political leadership. HIV prevalence rate among pregnant women is 17.0 percent.

1998: The activist group Treatment Action Campaign (TAC) is founded to campaign for the rights of people living with HIV and to demand access to HIV treatment in South Africa. Deputy President Thabo Mbeki launches the Partnership against AIDS, admitting that 1,500 HIV infections are occurring every day.

1999: HIV prevalence rate among pregnant women is 22.4 percent.

2000: The Department of Health outlines a five-year plan to combat AIDS, HIV, and other sexually transmitted diseases, with the National AIDS Council set up to oversee these developments. At the International AIDS Conference in Durban, the speech by the new South African president, Thabo Mbeki, avoids any reference to HIV and instead focuses on the problem of poverty, fueling suspicions that he sees poverty rather than HIV as the main cause of AIDS. President Mbeki consults a number of dissident scientists who reject the link between HIV and AIDS.

2001: Multinational drug companies withdraw a lawsuit against South Africa that would have prevented creation of cheaper, generic versions of patented AIDS drugs. HIV prevalence rate among pregnant women is 24.8 percent.

2002: South Africa's High Court orders the government to make the drug nevirapine available to pregnant women to help prevent mother-to-child transmission of HIV. Despite international drug companies' offers of free or cheap ARV drugs, the Health Department remains hesitant about providing treatment for people with HIV.

2003: In November, the government approves a plan to make ART available at no charge. Phase 1 of the first human clinical trial for a HIV vaccine is launched in Durban and Soweto. HIV prevalence rate among pregnant women is 27.9 percent.

2004: The government's ART program begins in Gauteng province in March, followed shortly afterward in other provinces.

2005: At least one service point for AIDS-related care and treatment has been established in all fifty-three districts in the country by March, meeting the government's 2003 target. However, the number of people receiving antiretroviral drugs is well behind targets. HIV prevalence rate among pregnant women is 30.2 percent.

2006: International AIDS experts call for the resignation of Health Minister Manto Tshabalala-Msimang after she openly promotes the use of garlic and beetroot as an alternative treatment for HIV at the sixteenth International AIDS Conference, in Toronto. Criticism of the government's response to AIDS heightens, with UN Special Envoy Stephen Lewis attacking the government as "obtuse, dilatory and negligent"[12] about treatment for AIDS. At the end of the year, the government announces a draft framework to tackle AIDS and pledges to improve access to antiretroviral drugs.

2007: The KwaZulu-Natal Department of Health charged Colin Pfaff with misconduct for providing dual antiretroviral prophylactic therapy to HIV-infected mothers. Dual therapy, recommended by WHO since August 2006, is more than twice as effective than monotherapy in lowering the risk of mother-to-child transmission. After being faced with significant pressure from local and global HIV activists, the country's health ministry revised its guidelines in February 2008 to include dual therapy, and charges against Dr. Pfaff were dropped.

2008: President Kgalema Motlanthe, on the first day of his presidency, removes Health Minister Manto Tshabalala-Msimang from office. A Harvard study estimates that 365,000 premature deaths could have been prevented in South Africa between 2000 and 2005, had the government provided ART to AIDS patients and provided treatment to HIV-infected pregnant women to prevent transmission to their infants. The new Minister of Health, Barbara Hogan, declares: "The era of denialism is over completely in South Africa."[13]

2009: HIV-infected Judge Edwin Cameron is appointed to South Africa's highest court. Judge Cameron was the first government official to disclose that he was HIV-positive.

Source: Adapted from AVERT, an International HIV and AIDS Charity. History of HIV and AIDS in South Africa. (http://www.avert.org/africa-aids-timeline.htm and http://www.avert.org/history-aids-south-africa.htm)

for the former apartheid government, it was viewed as a betrayal by the new democratic government. Nongovernmental organizations (NGOS; see the glossary) such as TAC, the Treatment Action Campaign, spearheaded campaigns for more access to treatment, lower drug prices, improved care, and a more effective policy on HIV/AIDS.

TAC, the most celebrated HIV advocacy group in the world, played a central role in combating the South African government's denial of HIV's impact. Founded in Cape Town in 1998 by Zackie Achmat, TAC campaigned for universal access to affordable ART and actions to support prevention and elimination of all new HIV infections. The organization has focused on social mobilization through treatment literacy and raising awareness of the constitutional right to healthcare.[14] TAC obtained a court order requiring the South African government to distribute nevirapine for the prevention of mother-to-child transmission. It successfully pressured pharmaceutical companies into lowering the cost of ART and was able to force the South African government to provide ART to the public. More than an advocacy group, it is credited with being a social movement that has successfully influenced policy formation and program implementation. It continues to work today, demanding expansion in prevention of mother-to-child transmission (PMTCT; see the glossary) protocols, advocating for community-based treatment of multidrug-resistant TB (MDR TB; see the glossary), and pressuring pharmaceutical companies to make new therapies, such as the HPV vaccine, more accessible.

In October 2003, the South African government finally committed to providing free ART to any person who qualified for treatment. Prior to this time, ART had been available only through private medical insurance, NGOS, or out-of-pocket payment. However, ART did not reach the public healthcare system until March 2004. Access to treatment continues to be a major barrier in the care of HIV-infected South Africans. The number of HIV-infected people able to access treatment has risen from fewer than 2,000 in 2003 to approximately 371,731 patients in 2007. Still, nearly half a million more people are estimated to be in need of ART. It is estimated that over 117,000 people are on waiting lists at public hospitals.[15]

Currently, ART can be initiated only by doctors. Given the scarcity of doctors, particularly in rural areas, this policy has significantly hindered the rollout of ART across the country. There are currently efforts to restructure prescribing practices for ART to make it a nurse-centered program. While this is an attractive idea, the number of nurses in the public sector (10 nurses per 10,000 uninsured persons) would still not be enough to meet the demand. In addition, the overall lack of health manpower is compounded by the deaths of HIV-infected healthcare workers. In 2002, it was estimated that 16 percent of health care workers were HIV-infected.[16]

The HIV/AIDS epidemic in South Africa has touched and destabilized every facet of life. With the disproportionate loss of working-age adults to HIV, many households' resources are stretched beyond limits. Entire families may rely on a single disability grant of $106 per month to feed as many as ten people. With inadequate government resources limiting medical care for HIV, few resources are left to address the social and economic impacts of the disease. As a result, families and communities have relied significantly on community-based organizations (CBOS; see the glossary), faith-based organizations (FBOS; see the glossary), and local and international NGOS to provide the services and support lacking from government programs. These organizations engage in education, advocacy, training, research, welfare and health service provision, orphan care, counseling, and other activities, and are integral to the comprehensive care of HIV-infected patients and their families.[17]

Tuberculosis

Fueled by the HIV epidemic, the incidence of TB in South Africa has skyrocketed in the past two decades. South Africa now ranks second in the world in incidence of TB. The current annual incidence rate of TB in the country is 940 cases per 100,000 people, up from 306 cases per 100,000 in 1990. HIV co-infection vastly increases the potential for an individual to progress to active TB. Although approximately one-third of the world's population is infected with *Mycobacterium tuberculosis*, the bacillus that causes TB (see the glossary), 90 percent of people will never manifest active disease given an adequate immune system. However, in the setting of HIV infection, the risk for TB reactivation increases nearly tenfold, to an annual risk of from 7 percent to 12 percent.[18] Additionally, HIV-infected individuals are more likely to progress to active disease following initial exposure to TB.[19] Given that nearly 20 percent of South Africa's population is HIV-infected, increasing the risk for progressing to active TB, and the fact that TB is propagated through airborne transmission, an epidemic of TB/HIV co-infection in South Africa was inevitable.

Although South Africa contains only 0.7 percent of the world's population, 28 percent of the world's cases of TB/HIV co-infection are found in the country. At least 40 percent of all new TB cases in South Africa are HIV co-infected;[20] in certain areas, the co-infection rate is as high as 80 percent.

While the two diseases are inextricably linked, the care provided to co-infected patients continues to be disjointed. Typically, HIV-infected patients are followed by the ART clinic, which is entirely separate from the TB clinic. Patients receive their medications separately, often having to wait hours in line to receive their ART only to walk over to another clinic to wait for their TB treatment. This separate care model results in redundancies in staff efforts and laboratory tests, and in fragmented care. While the government supports integrated HIV and TB care, TB and HIV programs continue to be separate, parallel systems, and patients continue to suffer complications of both diseases while never receiving the comprehensive attention they need.

South Africa has by far the most advanced healthcare infrastructure of all African nations, and the greatest capacity for extensive disease surveillance and control. However, its TB cure rate of 58 percent is one of the lowest among the ten countries with the highest TB burden. This has undoubtedly contributed to the emergence of MDR TB and extensively drug-resistant TB (XDR TB; see the glossary) in South Africa.

The Tugela Ferry Care and Research Collaboration, TF CaRes, is an international group of healthcare professionals focusing on epidemiological and operational research studies to improve care for HIV and TB in the rural, resource-limited setting of Tugela Ferry, in KwaZulu-Natal. Initially, TF CaRes began with an operational research study to examine the feasibility, safety, and effectiveness of integrating TB treatment and ART for TB-HIV co-infected patients.[21] This study demonstrated that integration of TB and HIV care improved survival and outcomes for both diseases.

The TB-HIV integration study also provided the first clues into the unrecognized, rapidly emerging, drug-resistant TB epidemic that now exists throughout South Africa. In 2006, our research group identified a large cohort of 221 MDR and 53 XDR TB patients at our study site in Tugela Ferry. Prior to 2006, it was thought that patients with MDR TB represented less than 2 percent of all new cases of TB in South Africa. However, our study revealed that 39 percent of all sputum-positive TB cultures were MDR TB, and 6 percent were XDR TB.[22] Of particular concern was the fact that the majority of XDR TB patients had never been previously treated for TB, suggesting transmission of drug-resistant TB strains as the underlying cause. These results raised significant alarm nationally and globally, as it became apparent that MDR and XDR TB were far more prevalent in South Africa than previously recognized. In response to these findings and to the resulting media coverage, the government, with help from WHO, directed over $200 million dollars toward the diagnosis and treatment of MDR TB. Hopefully, this new infusion of financial resources, along with heightened awareness of drug-resistant TB and TB-HIV co-infection will begin to turn the tide on the long-neglected TB epidemic in South Africa.

Diabetes and Cardiovascular Disease

The impact of diabetes and cardiovascular disease on morbidity and mortality in Africa is underappreciated. There is very little research in this field, as scientific efforts in this region have historically focused on infectious and communicable diseases. Not surprisingly though, the major risk factors for diabetes in South Africa are similar to those in the United States: urbanization, obesity, and physical inactivity. While Africa is often portrayed in the media as one homogeneous entity plagued by famine, disease, and malnourishment, the reality is that the continent is culturally and economically very diverse, and disease patterns remind us of this. No African country better embodies this cultural, economic, and health diversity than South Africa. In the past, it had been wealthier ethnic populations—whites and Indians—who traditionally suffered from diabetes and cardiovascular disease; now a growing proportion of the black population is also afflicted with these diseases.

Urbanization, with its related changes in work and transportation practices, has led to physical inactivity and obesity. While the prevalence of obesity in sub-Saharan Africa as a whole is only 2.5 percent, obesity is a well-established norm in South Africa. It is estimated that 31 percent of South African women are obese.[23]

A number of factors play a role in the prevalence of obesity. Because of its relative wealth and established agricultural economy, South Africa does not suffer the same issues of food insecurity as do many other African countries. A greater proportion of the population has sufficient access to food, and because of the stable agricultural system, food production remains relatively constant. Additionally, the country's welfare system provides grants for impoverished families, which further improves access to food. Although these grants are modest, their impact is substantial in diminishing the population at risk for malnutrition and starvation. This is a benefit not enjoyed by most other African countries. Cultural perceptions may also play a role in the social acceptance of obesity. A larger body size is perceived as a sign of affluence, while weight loss may be negatively associated with the wasting seen in AIDS.

With obesity increasing, the estimated prevalence of diabetes in South Africa (5.3 percent to 8 percent of the population) is much higher than other nations in the region (approximately 3.1 percent).[24] Microvascular complications, such as foot ulcers, neuropathies and retinopathy, are the most common consequences of diabetic disease in South Africa. In most cases the damage is irreversible, as patients present late in their disease course. Macrovascular complications, such as heart disease and stroke, are less common in diabetics of African descent than those of European or mixed ancestry. The reasons for this difference are not well studied, but it is believed that other risk factors for ischemic heart disease such as smoking, hypercholesterolemia, and hypertension are less common in rural, traditional black populations. We do know that black South Africans, when compared to white South Africans, have lower triglyceride levels and lower rates of smoking.[25] However, urban black South Africans show a higher incidence of these risk factors when compared to their rural counterparts. It is likely that with urbanization and economic development, the risk for heart disease will continue to rise in the black population.

Diabetes and cardiovascular diseases pose challenges to the South African healthcare system, which has been built around the management of acute rather than chronic care. To manage the increasing costs of diabetes and other chronic diseases, the healthcare system will have to incorporate better screening and management training for healthcare workers, supply appropriate equipment to facilitate early screening at clinics, and improve health education for the population at large.

Violence and Injury

Although the 1994 transition to a democratic society was a model of nonviolent change in power, it took decades of state-sponsored oppression, political violence, and protest to bring South Africa to that moment. The apartheid regime fueled a culture of violence through a deliberate disintegration of ethnic and social communities, the breakdown of traditional family structure, and the creation of vast economic and health disparities that persist today.

There are an estimated 60,000 non-natural deaths in South Africa each year, accounting for 12 percent of all mortality in the country.[26] Violence and road traffic accidents are the leading causes of non-natural deaths and together make injury the third major cause of mortality in South Africa.[27] Intentional and unintentional injuries are the second leading cause of all disability-adjusted life-years, after HIV/AIDS. The major contributors to the injury burden are homicide—largely from firearms—(45 percent), transportation-related incidents (27 percent), suicide (10 percent), and other unintentional injuries such as burns and poisonings (10 percent). The country's mortality rates from homicide, road traffic accidents, and suicides far exceed global averages, and younger, poorer South African populations, such as those in the townships, are disproportionately affected.

Gender-based violence is also a significant form of violence in the community. The rate of female homicides, 31.7 per 100,000 women, is seven times greater than the global average. Fifty percent of South African women who are killed by a known perpetrator are killed by an intimate partner. Rape is also grossly underreported, but studies have shown the prevalence of reported rapes to be 1,300 per 100,000 women.[28] Drugs, alcohol, and easy availability of firearms are all major factors contributing to violent injuries.

An issue receiving increasing attention today is the problem of violence in South African schools. It appears that schools both perpetrate violence and reflect themes of crime and violence in the greater society.[29] Children create games in response to violence they observe, such as "rape me rape me," where they play-act incidents of sexual assault. Attending school is a particular risk for female students, who may be sexually assaulted both on the long journeys to and from school and by teachers once at school. Twenty percent of all sexual assaults on female students occur at school, with 9 percent being committed by teachers.[30] The presence of physical violence has increased with the increasing presence of knives, handguns, and other weapons on school premises. While community issues such as substance abuse, poverty, and community violence fuel school violence, aspects of the school environment itself— deteriorating facilities and the use of physical punishment by teaching personnel—contribute to the degradation of the learning environment.

It is difficult to quantify the health and social impacts of violence, since the effects extend beyond just the victim. In South Africa, as in all societies, the true extent of the problem of violence is underestimated.

Conclusion

South Africa is simultaneously the easiest and most difficult African country to live in. In this English-speaking country with impressive racial diversity and an abundance of modern amenities, you are often reminded of home. However, its unique history has pervaded every aspect of life, and though it may not be immediately apparent, it's not far below the surface.

South Africa has many of the modern amenities that we enjoy at home (often at lower prices). Modern European-style cafes and art galleries line the cities and suburbs, giving you the opportunity to have a good cappuccino or visit an art exhibit. However, if you will be working in global health in South Africa, your work will likely be with a disenfranchised population. This means that you will face the harsh juxtaposition of shuttling between the posh neighborhood where you live or spend the weekends and where you work—likely a community of mud homes without running water, sanitation, or electricity. This disparity is further exacerbated by the devastating impact that HIV has had. Patients are often far sicker than their counterparts in the West, making it difficult to reconcile how part of society can have wealth that rivals that of U.S. and European upper classes, yet the communities you're working with suffer from inadequate resources, like those typically seen in the poorest countries. This disconnect may bring out feelings of frustration or anger, which you must recognize and address in order to remain productive.

South Africa is full of fascinating cities and astoundingly beautiful places. Exploring them should be a central part of your experience. However, we must also provide a message of caution. South Africa is a dangerous place whether you're in the city or in rural areas. It has one of the highest rates of violent crimes in the world, particularly rape, which is a very real threat to any woman working in the country. Traveling alone, whether you are a man or woman, is not recommended, and you must be very cautious about using public transportation. As a visitor less familiar with where you're going, you would be an easy target for mugging on public transportation.

On the other hand, in South Africa it is hard not to blend in. While in other African countries, a white or Asian health worker might stand out, in South Africa you will hardly garner a second glance, given the local racial diversity. However, because of the country's history of apartheid, you may find yourself becoming acutely aware of race, what "category" people will perceive you as, and how they will react to you. Generally, as a foreigner you are rarely a target of racial bias, but the presence of race becomes more of a reality than you may be used to at home.

One of the more difficult cultural practices to accept is the use of traditional medicine, called *muti*. While traditional healers often use innocuous herbs, they also use hazardous concoctions, sometimes prescribing battery acid for enemas or treating TB with mixtures that can cause liver damage. Patients very commonly seek care from traditional healers before seeing a medical doctor, so it is important to elicit this history from your patients. Local beliefs significantly affect those doing HIV work specifically. Misconceptions are pervasive (for instance, the belief that Americans brought HIV to South Africa). During the Mbeki administration, misconceptions were deliberately created and promoted by government leaders (for instance, that the CIA and Western drug companies promote the belief that HIV causes AIDS to increase the sales of anti-HIV drugs). Unfortunately, the legacy of such misconceptions remains in many communities. Researchers are often perceived as gathering information clandestinely for malicious purposes, despite the fact that numerous research groups and NGOs have been working in South Africa to advance the understanding of HIV and improve its care.

While some of what we describe here presents challenges and the need to exercise caution when working in South Africa, many wonderful opportunities exist to substantially impact the health and lives of individuals and entire populations. It is a country with great need, but also the necessary resources and infrastructure to make a difference.

In summary, politics, economics, and public health in modern South Africa are inextricably linked to the previous policies of the apartheid era. Nonetheless, South Africa has emerged from the history of an oppressive, segregationist regime into one of the most stable, vibrant, and multicultural democracies on the African continent. Much progress has been made in racially integrating society, but many additional challenges remain. South Africa remains economically dichotomous, mostly along racial lines, with both a first world and a third world existing simultaneously. Efforts to eliminate the inequities between racial groups have been partially successful in creating an elite, black upper class and growing middle class, but further efforts are needed to address the needs of the poor. Public health policies have now shifted to address the basic health needs of the majority of the population, while trying to maintain the high quality of care that existed previously for the upper-class white population. In the future, economic development is likely to bring a new set of growing public health challenges as the prevalence of chronic, degenerative diseases increases. At the same time, pressing public health issues, such as the explosive HIV epidemic, will impact the country's economy if greater efforts are not made to address them more effectively and vigorously. The search for answers to public health problems in South Africa will have to take into account the economic and political factors influencing them, since only multifaceted solutions are likely to be successful.

COUNTRY DATA : SOUTH AFRICA

Millennium Development Goal indicators are italicized.

TABLE 7.1 : POPULATION AND HUMAN DEVELOPMENT

POPULATION	
Total	49.0 million
Population growth rate	0.28%
Net migration rate/1,000 population	−0.13
Urban	61%
Rural	39%
AGE STRUCTURE	
0–14 years	28.2%
15–64 years	65.8%
65+ years	5.4%
Median age (years)	24.4
MAJOR ETHNIC GROUPS	
Black African	79.0%
White	9.6%
Colored	8.9%
Indian/Asian	2.5%
RELIGIONS	
Christian	79.7%
Muslim	1.5%
Other	3.7%
None	15.1%
HUMAN DEVELOPMENT	
Human Development Index	0.683
Human Development rank[a]	125th
Freedom House Index	Free
Political Rights score[b]	2
Civil Liberties score[b]	2
Human Poverty Index	23.5
Human Poverty rank[c]	121st

Notes: [a]out of 179 countries; [b]1 = most free; 7 = least free; [c]out of 177 countries

TABLE 7.2 : **GOVERNMENT AND ECONOMY**

GOVERNMENT	
Independence (union of 4 British colonies)	31 May 1910
Republic declared	31 May 1961
Majority rule	27 Apr. 1994
Type of government	Republic
Voting rights	Age 18, universal
CAPITAL	Pretoria
CURRENCY	Rand (ZAR)
ECONOMY	
Gross Domestic Product (GDP) (in PPP US $)	489.7 billion
Annual GDP growth	2.8%
GDP per capita (in US $)	$10,000
Gini Index	65
Population living below PPP $1/day	26.2%
External debt service as % of GDP	2.0
Public debt as % of GDP	31.6
Official development assistance (ODA)- per capita (in US $)	$15.5
Foreign direct investment as % of GDP	2.6
LABOR FORCE	
In agriculture	9%
In industry	26%
In services	65%
Unemployment rate	22.9%

TABLE 7.3 : **GEOGRAPHY AND ENVIRONMENT**

LAND COMPOSITION

Land area	1,219,090 sq. km. (470,693 sq. mi.)
Size comparison	Slightly less than twice the size of Texas
Terrain	Vast interior plateau rimmed by rugged hills and narrow coastal plain; 2,798-km. (1,738-mi.) coastline
Ecological hazards	Prolonged droughts

LAND USE AND RESOURCES

Permanent crop land	0.79%
Arable land	12.1%
Agricultural products	Corn, wheat, sugarcane, fruit, vegetables, livestock, wool, dairy products
Natural resources	Uranium, diamonds, platinum, natural gas, gold, chromium, antimony, coal, iron ore, manganese, nickel, tin

ENVIRONMENTAL ISSUES

Lack of large rivers or lakes, need for water conservation control measures, water use outstripping supply, acid rain, soil erosion, desertification

INFRASTRUCTURE

Population with access to improved water source	*93%*
Population using improved sanitation	*59%*
Roadways unpaved	79.7%

TABLE 7.4 : **HEALTH**

LIFE, BIRTH, AND DEATH

Life expectancy at birth (male/female)	49.8/48.1
Birth rate/1,000 population	19.93
Death rate/1,000 population	16.94
Infant mortality rate/1,000 live births	*44.42*

PERSONNEL AND INFRASTRUCTURE

Physicians/100,000 population	77
Hospital beds/10,000 population	28

Total expenditure on health per capita (PPP US $) $748

Public expenditure on health as % of GDP   3.5

Most common vector-borne diseases   Malaria, Crimean Congo hemorrhagic fever

Most common food- and water-borne diseases   Bacterial diarrhea, hepatitis A, typhoid fever, schistosomiasis

TB incidence/100,000 population   *940*

TB prevalence/100,000 population   *998*

New TB cases HIV-positive   44%

New TB cases multidrug- resistant (MDR)   1.8%

1-year-olds fully immunized against TB   99%

Estimated malaria cases annually   18,000–55,000

Malaria death rate/100,000 population   0.02

HIV prevalence rate in adults   *18.1%*

AIDS deaths in adults annually   *350,000*

People living with HIV   5.7 million

AIDS orphans   1.4 million

Fertility rate (children born per woman)   2.38

Contraceptive prevalence rate (married women 15–49)   *60.3%*

Maternal mortality rate/100,000 births   *400*

Lifetime risk of maternal death, 1 in: *110*

Births attended by skilled birth attendant   *92%*

Mortality rate of children < 5/1,000 live births   *59*

1-year-olds immunized against measles   *83%*

Children < 5 using insecticide-treated bed nets   *NA*

Children < 5 with fever treated with antimalarial drugs   *NA*

Newborns protected against tetanus   72%

Children < 5 underweight for age   *11.5%*

Children < 5 under height for age   *31%*

Population undernourished   *NA*

TABLE 7.5 : **LANGUAGE, EDUCATION, AND LITERACY**

LANGUAGES	
IsiZulu	23.8%
IsiXhosa	17.6%
Afrikaans	13.3%
Sepedi	9.4%
English	8.2%
Setswana	8.2%
Other	19.5%
LITERACY	
Adult literacy rate (population age 15+ who can read and write)	86.4%
EXPENDITURE	
Public expenditure on education as % of GDP	5.4
EDUCATION	
Net enrollment in primary education[d]	91.0%
School life expectancy, in years (male/female)[e]	13/13

[d]Net enrollment rate in primary education is measured as the number of children of official primary school age who are enrolled in primary education as a percentage of children in the official primary school age population.

[e]School life expectancy is the total number of years of school (from primary through tertiary education) that a child can expect to receive.

Principal Sources for Data in Appendix Tables 7.1–7.5

Central Intelligence Agency, *The World Factbook* (https://www.cia.gov/library/publications/the-world-factbook/).

UNDP Human Development Report, 2007/2008, available at: www.hdrstats.undp.org.

UN Millennium Development Goals Indicators Database, available at www.mdgs.un.org.

UNICEF. The State of the World's Children 2009. Available at: www.data.un.org.

WHO. Global Tuberculosis Control. Country Profile: South Africa. WHO Report 2009.

NOTES

1. The French villages are populated by descendents of French Huguenots who arrived in South Africa in the seventeenth century, and established farming villages and vineyards which still stand today in the Western Cape region of the

country. The minstrel carnival is a minstrel festival that takes place in January every year in Cape Town.

2. For an example, see the description of post-independence attempts at socialism in the chapter on Tanzania.

3. The Freedom Charter, adopted at the Congress of the People, Kliptown, South Africa, 26 June 1955 (http://www.sahistory.org.za/pages/governence -projects/freedom-charter/07_charter.htm).

4. Nelson Mandela, "Inaugural Address," Pretoria, South Africa, 9 May 1994 (http://www.speech-topics-help.com/nelson-mandelas-inaugural-speech .htmlhttp), or (http://www.wsu.edu:8080/~wldciv/world_civ_reader/world_civ _reader_2/mandela.html).

5. United Nations. International Convention on the Suppression and Punishment of the Crime of Apartheid, New York, 30 November 1973 (http://zvon.org/ law/r/apartheid.html);Truth and Reconciliation Commission of South Africa Report, Volume 6, Cape Town, South Africa, March 2003 (www.info.gov.za/ otherdocs/2003/trc/rep.pdf).

6. Chris McGreal."There's Racism, but Not in Public," *The Guardian*, 7 March 2008 (http://www.guardian.co.uk/world/2008/mar/07/southafrica.race).

7. Statistics South Africa, "General Household Survey 2007" (10 July 2008; http://www.statssa.gov.za/publications/statsdownload.asp?ppn=P0318&SCH= 4187).

8. M. T. Bassett et al., "HIV Infection in Urban Males in Zimbabwe," paper presented at the Sixth International Conference on AIDS, San Francisco, 20-24 June 1990; M. N. Lurie et al., "Who Infects Whom? HIV-1 Concordance and Discordance among Migrant and Non-migrant Couples in South Africa," *AIDS* 17, no. 15 (2003): 2245-52.

9. Lurie et al., "Who Infects Whom?"

10. Although symbolically considered self-governing states, health systems in the homelands were effectively controlled by the Department of National Health and Population Development. The homelands' characterization as autonomous entities allowed the South African government to avoid its responsibilities there and blame the poor health and health services on homeland authorities.

11. Cedric De Beer, *The South African Disease: Apartheid Health and Health Services* (Johannesburg: South African Research Services, 1984).

12. Remarks by Stephen Lewis, UN Special Envoy for HIV/AIDS in Africa, to the Closing Session of the XVI International AIDS Conference, Toronto, Canada, (18 August 2006; http://www.kaisernetwork.org/health_cast/hcast_index.cfm ?display=detail&hc=1814). Then choose Keynote Address. Stephen Lewis.

13. Barbara Hogan, quoted in Celia Dugger, "Study Cites Toll of AIDS Policy in South Africa," *The New York Times*, 25 November 2008.

14. For more information, see TAC's website (http://www.tac.org.za).

15. UNAIDS, "Epidemiological Fact Sheet on HIV and AIDS. South Africa .2008 Update." Geneva, UNAIDs/WHO Working Group on HIV/AIDS and STI Surveillance, (September 2008; http://www.unaids.org/en/CountryResponses/ Countries/south_africa.asp, then go to Epidemiological Fact Sheet on HIV and AIDS, 2008 to download full report.).

16. O. Shisana et al., "HIV/AIDS Prevalence among South African Health Workers," *South African Medical Journal* 94 (2004): 846-50.

17. Given the reliance on CBOs, FBOs, and NGOs in South Africa for services related to HIV/AIDS and TB, if you are going to South Africa you will want to become familiar with some of the following key organizations and related medical research institutions in the country: Africa Centre for Health and Population Studies, AIDS Consortium, AIDS Foundation of South Africa, AIDS Law Project, Aram Institute for Health Research, Centre for the AIDS Program of Research in South Africa, Desmond Tutu HIV Foundation, Desmond Tutu TB Centre at Stellenbosch University, Enhancing Care Initiative, McCord Hospital, Médicins sans Frontières, South African Medical Research Council, and TAC.

18. P. A. Selwyn et al., "A Prospective Study of the Risk of Tuberculosis among Intravenous Drug Users with Human Immunodeficiency Virus Infection," *New England Journal of Medicine* 320, no. 9 (1989): 545-50.

19. C. L. Daley et al., "An Outbreak of Tuberculosis with Accelerated Progression among Persons Infected with the Human Immunodeficiency Virus: An Analysis Using Restriction-fragment-length Polymorphisms," *New England Journal of Medicine* 326, no. 4 (1992): 231-35.

20. World Health Organization, "Global Tuberculosis Control 2008: Surveillance, Planning, Financing" (2008; http://www.who.int/tb/publications/global _report/2008/pdf/report_without_annexes.pdf).

21. N. R. Gandhi et al., "Successful Integration of Tuberculosis and HIV Treatment in Rural South Africa: The Sizonq'oba Study," *Journal of Acquired Immune Deficiency Syndromes* 50, no. 1 (2009): 37-43.

22. N. R. Gandhi et al., "Extensively Drug-resistant Tuberculosis as a Cause of Death in Patients Co-infected with Tuberculosis and HIV in a Rural Area of South Africa," *Lancet* 368 (2006): 1575-80.

23. C. Monteiro et al., "Obesity and Inequities in Health in the Developing World," *International Journal of Obesity* 28, no. 9 (2004): 1181-86.

24. A. Motala et al., "Diabetes and Other Disorders of Glyceamia in a Rural South African Community: Prevalence and Associated Risk Factors." *Diabetes Care* 31, no. 9 (September 2008): 1783-1788 (http://care.diabetesjournals.org/ content/31/9/1783.full).

25. W. J. Kalk and B. I. Joffe, "Differences in Coronary Heart Disease Prevalence and Risk Factors in African and White Patients with Type 2 Diabetes," *Diabetes Research and Clinical Practice* 77, no. 1 (2007): 107-12.

26. National Injury Mortality Surveillance System, "Violence and Injury" (2005; http://www.sahealthinfo.org/violence/nimss.htm).

27. A useful perspective on traffic accidents as a significant cause of mortality in Africa is provided in the chapter on Ghana.

28. R. Jewkes and N. Abrahams, "The Epidemiology of Rape and Sexual Coercion in South Africa: An Overview," *Social Science & Medicine* 55 (2002): 1231–44.

29. South African Human Rights Commission, "Report on School-Based Violence," Pretoria, South Africa, 12 March 2008. (http://edulibpretoria.wordpress .com/downloads/, then search under 2008 publications for SAHRC report on School-Based Violence for downloadable chapters of the full report).

30. Ibid.

SUGGESTED READING

Apartheid and History of South Africa

Krog, Antjie. *Country of My Skull: Guilt, Sorrow and the Limits of Forgiveness in the New South Africa*. New York: Times, 1999.

Malan, Rian. *My Traitor's Heart: A South African Exile Returns to Face His Country, His Tribe, and His Conscience*. New York: Atlantic Monthly, 1990.

Mandela, Nelson. *Long Walk to Freedom: The Autobiography of Nelson Mandela* (paperback) Boston: Back Bay, 1995. "Long walk to freedom: the autobiography of Nelson Mandela. 1st ed. Published/Created, Boston: Little, Brown, c1994.

Thompson, Leonard. *A History of South Africa*. New Haven, Conn.: Yale University Press, 2001.

Fiction

Paton, Alan. *Cry the Beloved Country*. (paperback) New York: Scribner, 1987.

HIV/AIDS and Tuberculosis

Davies, G. R., M. Pillay, A. W. Sturm, and D. Wilkinson. "Emergence of Multi-drug Resistant Tuberculosis in a Community-based Directly Observed Treatment Programme in Rural South Africa." *International Journal of Tuberculosis and Lung Disease* 3, no. 9 (1999): 799–804.

DeRiemer, K., et al. "Does DOTS Work in Populations with Drug-resistant Tuberculosis?" *Lancet* 365, no. 9466 (2005): 1239–45.

Friedland, Gerald. "Utility of Tuberculosis Directly Observed Therapy Programs as Sites for Access to and Provision of Antiretroviral Therapy in Resource-Limited Countries." *Clinical Infectious Diseases* 38, Supplement 5 (2004): S421–28.

Friedland, G., G. Churchyard, and F. Nardell, eds. "TB/HIV Coinfection."

Supplement to *Journal of Infectious Diseases*, 196 (Suppl. 3), August 2007. [A collection of twelve articles addressing issues in TB/HIV coinfection.]

Gandhi, N. R., et al. "Successful Integration of Tuberculosis and HIV Treatment in Rural South Africa: The Sizonq'oba Study." *Journal of Acquired Immune Deficiency Syndromes* 50, no. 1 (2009): 37–43.

Gellman, Barton. A series of articles in *The Washington Post*, including: "Death Watch: The Global Response to AIDS in Africa. World Shunned Signs of the Coning Plague," July 2000 (http://www.washingtonpost.com/wp-dyn/content/article/2006/06/09/AR2006060901326.html); "A Turning Point That Left Millions Behind: Drug Discounts Benefit Few While Protecting Pharmaceutical Companies' Profits," 28 December 2000 (http://www.washingtonpost.com/wp-dyn/content/article/2006/06/09/AR2006060901310.html); "An Unequal Calculus of Life and Death: As Millions Perished in Pandemic, Firms Debated Access to Drugs; Players in the Debate Over Drug Availability and Pricing," 27 December 2000 (http://www.washingtonpost.com/wp-dyn/content/article/2006/06/09/AR2006060901287.html)

Karim, Salim S. Abdool, et al. "Implementing Antiretroviral Therapy in Resource-constrained Settings: Opportunities and Challenges in Integrating HIV and Tuberculosis Care." *AIDS* 18, no. 7 (2004): 975–79.

Karim, S. S. Abdool, and Q. Abdool Karim, eds. *HIV/AIDS in South Africa*. Cape Town: Cambridge University Press, 2005.

Power, Samantha. "Letter from South Africa: The AIDS Rebel." (Abstract) *New Yorker*, 19 May 2003, 54 (http://www.newyorker.com/archive/2003/05/19/030519fa_fact_power).

Wilson, D. "Diagnosing HIV-Associated Tuberculosis." *Southern African Journal of HIV Medicine* 6, no. 2 (2005): 23–26.

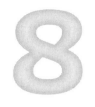

LISA V. ADAMS

HELGA NABURI

RICHARD WADDELL

TANZANIA

Tanzania: Cradle of Humankind

In 1959, in the Olduvai Gorge in western Tanganyika, as the country was known during its period of British occupation, the famed archae- ologists Louis and Mary Leakey discovered an intact human fossil skull and other bones dating back 1.85 million years which they described as *Homo habilis* or Handy Man. This finding generated the belief that this region of Eastern Africa was the cradle of humankind.[1]

Today, Tanzania is an independent, democratic country in East Africa. Immediately south of the equator, it is bordered by the Indian Ocean on the east; Kenya and Uganda on the north; Rwanda, Burundi, and the Democratic Republic of the Congo on the west; and Zambia, Malawi, and Mozambique on the south.

Tanzania is well known for its natural splendor. Travelers come for the adventure of going on safari in its famous national parks and game preserves such as the Serengeti—where lions, wildebeest, elephants, gazelles, zebras, and hippos live in natural balance—or to climb Mt. Kilimanjaro, the highest peak in Africa. The magnificent white sand beaches on the islands of Zanzibar and Pemba also lure visitors. With so much natural beauty and a burgeoning tourist industry, Tanzania is becoming a common tourist destination, no longer reserved for youth- ful backpackers or intrepid explorers.

Tanzania is much more than its offerings of wildlife safaris, mountain trekking, and exotic beaches, however. Its strengths include a peace- ful, democratic system of governance and a relatively united populace, notable in a region often troubled by tribal conflicts and political instability. While more than 120 tribes live within its borders, each with its own language, most Tanzanians feel a strong national identity. To promote unity across tribal groups, Kiswahili was made an official national language in 1984; it is the language used in social discourse, business, politics and primary education. Tanzania's political stability has allowed the country to experience several periods of economic growth since independence. Nonetheless, with a gross domestic product (GDP; see the glossary) of $1,300 per person, Tanzania ranks in the poorest 10 percent of the world's countries. It faces many health problems common to low-income countries in a tropical setting: unacceptably high morbidity and mortality from infectious diseases, and life-threatening conditions affecting maternal and child health—all made worse by a struggling healthcare infrastructure. Like many of its African neighbors, Tanzania has been losing its skilled and educated workforce to better paying positions in the United States, Europe, and South Africa—the so-called brain drain.

While travel guides will describe Tanzania's popular tourist destinations (which we encourage you to experience when you are in the country), our aim in this chapter is to introduce you to the country's health system, the critical health issues that Tanzanians face, and the many national and international agencies and programs at work in the country. Finally, we share some of our experiences, in the hope that what we have learned might help prepare you for global health and humanitarian work in Tanzania or elsewhere in Africa.

Historical Perspectives

Tanzania is a combination of Tanganyika, the name of the large mainland territory, and Zanzibar, the name of the archipelago northeast of Dar es Salaam, the country's largest and principal commercial city and its cultural and diplomatic capital. Tanzania was formed in 1964, following Tanganyika's independence from Britain in 1961 and Zanzibar's independence first from Britain in 1963 and then from the Sultan of Zanzibar in 1964 during the Zanzibar Revolution. In 1996, all government offices were transferred from Dar es Salaam to Dodoma, making it the country's political capital.[2]

The Leakey archaeological finds in western Tanzania suggest that this region has been inhabited since prehistoric times. Trading contacts existed between the East African coast and Arabia by the first century, followed by the Portuguese in the late fifteenth century and the French in the sixteenth, predominantly for slave trade and exploitation of natural resources such as ivory. Nineteenth-century German missionaries reached the Kilimanjaro region. The first British explorers in the area, Richard Burton and John Hanning Speke, traveled west to Lake Tanganyika and Lake Victoria in 1857-58, followed by the geographic explorers David Livingstone and Henry Morton Stanley. Early visitors to Zanzibar included the Persians, Hindus, Jews, Arabs, Phoenicians, and possibly the Assyrians.

Tanganyika (the mainland) was a German colony from the early 1880s until the end of World War I, when the League of Nations charter designated the area as a British mandate, and it was governed as a trust territory in the interests of the native inhabitants. The Zanzibar islands were under the rule of the sultanate of Oman at the time. One of Britain's first actions in Tanganyika was to abolish slavery. The British governor of Tanganyika, Sir Donald Cameron, worked out a plan that gave some authority to tribal leaders, involving them in local decision making through the Native Authority Ordinance of 1926. With a well-organized economy, this tolerant legislative system resulted in an increased number of educated Africans. However, during the worldwide economic depression of the 1930s, many of Cameron's programs were curtailed.[3] In 1947, the British government decided to put the mainland under a UN trusteeship, working in concert with the British Governor.

The transition to independence in Tanganyika was more or less peaceful. A good part of this can be attributed to Julius Nyerere, an intellectual and former schoolteacher who entered politics in the early 1950s. Elected president of the Tanganyika Africa Association in 1953, Nyerere transformed the organization from a social club into the politically oriented Tanganyika African National Union. The union's objective was to achieve national sovereignty for an independent Tanganyika. Following a series of constitutional and parliamentary changes through which the Governor effectively lost power, Nyerere became the country's first minister of British-administered Tanganyika in 1960, and continued as prime minister after independence in 1961. Shortly thereafter, he assumed the country's presidency and held that office until 1985.[4]

Nyerere immediately began to rebuild the country after its nearly 100 years of foreign rule, using a model of social and economic development that focused on *ujamaa* (Swahili for extended family or family-hood) and the fundamental African socioeconomic unit—the village. Nyerere's plan also entailed a commitment to pan-African socialism. Banks and many industries were nationalized. The initial results were positive: literacy increased, poverty was reduced, and medical services were strengthened by improved health education and disease treatment programs. As part of its socialist endeavors, Tanzania sought an alignment with China. Imported Chinese labor and the formation of collective farms forced relocation of many Tanzanians. The failure of these socialist experiments—together with an oil price spike, a drop in commodity prices in the 1970s, and a series of droughts—left the economy in turmoil by the 1980s.

The Tanzanian government agreed to accept conditional loans from the International Monetary Fund and underwent structural adjustments that resulted in sizable liquidation of the public sector, deregulation of financial and agricultural markets, and adjustments to healthcare models.[5] Through the mid-1990s, the country's GDP grew modestly, but poverty levels also increased.

Tanzania Today

Tanzania remains one of the world's poorest countries. In recent years it has been in the top tier of recipients of nonmilitary aid, especially for the treatment of HIV/AIDS and tuberculosis (TB). Recent public-sector and banking reforms and new legislative frameworks have spurred private-sector growth and nongovernmental investment.[6]

Tanzania's economy is largely based on agriculture, which accounts for more than 50 percent of its GDP, 85 percent of exports, and 80 percent of the workforce. Although 75 percent of the people live in rural areas, the population is unevenly distributed, ranging from one person per square kilometer (three per square mile) in the most arid regions, to 52 per square kilometer (133 per square mile) in the highlands, and 134 per square kilometer (347 per square mile) in Zanzibar. Unemployment is extremely high, unofficially it is estimated to be at about 67 percent.

The majority of Tanzanians have Bantu origins. Much of Zanzibar's African population came from the mainland, but one group (the Afro-Shirazis) may be the descendants of the early Persian traders. Only 1 percent of the total population is non-African. Data on religion were eliminated from government census reports after 1967, but religious leaders and sociologists estimate that Christians and Muslims each account for 30 percent to 35 percent of the mainland population (Muslims account for more than 99 percent of the population in Zanzibar), with the remainder following other faiths including indigenous religions, or being nonbelievers.[7]

Tanzania has a history of being a haven for refugees and asylum seekers. In 2007, the country was host to nearly 500,000 refugees, primarily from Burundi and the Democratic Republic of the Congo.[8] This acceptance of other nationals dates to President Nyerere's long and vociferous opposition to apartheid; indeed, he became known as the "conscience of black Africa" because of his active support for African liberation struggles. During the troubled years of Idi Amin's reign in Uganda, both Milton Obote, president of Uganda in 1966–71, and Yoweri Museveni, Uganda's current president, sought refuge in Tanzania. In October 1978, Amin invaded Tanzania, heavily bombing the Lake Victoria ports of Bukoba and Musoma. Nyerere assembled a people's militia, routed the Ugandan forces and took control of Uganda's capital Kampala, leading to Amin's eventual downfall. This effort to liberate Africa from dictatorship cost Tanzania an estimated $500 million, creating a harsh financial burden for the country.[9]

Since democracy was introduced in 1992, Tanzania has enjoyed a stable political and economic climate. Despite a severe drought in 2005, which significantly affected agricultural production, Tanzania's GDP has grown at a steady rate (7.1 percent in 2008), and inflation has remained in the single digits.[10] The current administration is focusing on infrastructure development, including expansion of the railway system to provide a gateway to East Africa, in the hope of creating an economic environment conducive to further investment and growth.

Tanzania's Healthcare System

The Ministry of Health and Social Welfare (MOHSW) is the government agency responsible for health. The MOHSW runs the main referral or consultant hospitals and health training schools, and oversees agencies with health-related responsibilities such as the Tanzania Food and Drug Authority, the Medical Stores Department (responsible for the procurement and distribution of pharmaceuticals), the National Institute for Medical Research, and the Tanzania Food and Nutrition Centre. The health policy aim in Tanzania is to improve the health and well-being of all citizens, with a focus on those at risk, and to encourage the health system to be more responsive to the needs of the people.[11]

Health services in Tanzania are delivered through the public sector, which includes the MOHSW and parastatal organizations (controlled wholly or in part by the government); the private sector; nongovernmental organizations (NGOS; see the glossary); and faith-based organizations (FBOS; see the glossary).

In the public system, health services are organized in a hierarchy from the national to the regional to the district levels. The regional medical officer is responsible for health services in the region and also coordinates and supervises activities at the district level. The district medical officer is responsible for health services carried out at district hospitals, health centers, and dispensaries.

The private sector (including both for-profit and not-for-profit entities) currently supplies about one-third of all health services in Tanzania. Private-sector organizations provide mainly curative health services, offering few preventive services. NGOS, FBOS, and other private-sector facilities are guided by MOHSW standards and protocols, and the MOHSW provides support by training their staffs, sometimes assigning its own personnel to these facilities, and providing medicines and vaccines.

A patient's route through the healthcare system follows a pyramidal pattern: patients are referred up the hierarchy from village health posts to dispensaries, local health centers, and district and regional hospitals. The structure of health services is as follows:[12]

> *Village health posts* are the most local level of healthcare delivery and essentially provide preventive services. Each post is staffed by two health workers from the community who have completed basic clinical training.
> *The dispensary* offers care to about 6,000 to 10,000 people and supervises the village health posts in its ward. Dispensaries are staffed by a clinical officer, nurse-midwife, maternal-child health aide, nurse assistant, and laboratory assistant.
> *A health center* offers care for 50,000 people, which is the typical population of one administrative division. Health centers are

staffed by a range of medical providers and include maternal and child health, laboratory, and pharmacy services.

Most districts have *a district hospital*; for those without one, the government helps finance a hospital from the NGO sector to serve this function. The district hospital offers diagnostic, laboratory, radiology, and surgical services, including emergency obstetric care. District hospitals are the first level of referral hospitals.

Regional hospitals provide a higher level of specialized care to a well-defined geographic area. They are staffed by general surgeons, adult and pediatric physicians, nurses, midwives, and public health staff.

Referral or consultant hospitals provide complex healthcare requiring advanced technology and highly skilled personnel. They are also teaching hospitals, serving as training sites for health service workers. The main referral and teaching hospitals in Tanzania are Muhimbili National Hospital, in Dar es Salaam; Kilimanjaro Christian Medical Centre, in Moshi; and Bugando Medical Centre, in Mwanza. Two other hospitals—Mbeya Hospital in Mbeya, and Mnazimmoja Hospital in Stone Town, Zanzibar—are referral hospitals but not teaching hospitals.

There is a range of additional health services, some of which may be unfamiliar to foreigners:

Private maternity homes work in close collaboration with the MOHSW's Reproductive Health and Child Health Programme to offer pediatric care, reproductive and family planning services, and—in some cases—services to prevent mother-to-child transmission of HIV.

Private clinics and pharmacies provide mostly curative services and are operated by FBOS and NGOS.

Voluntary counseling and testing facilities are stand-alone centers that provide HIV/AIDS counseling and testing services. They can be managed by the government, NGOS, FBOS, or private for-profit enterprises. Their services are now being integrated into primary care provided at general health facilities.

Through *home-based care* provided by NGOS or supervised community volunteers, chronically ill patients receive curative or psychological care in their homes.

Public health programs target specific diseases and promote preventive services. The central unit of each disease program is located in the MOHSW, with coordinators at the regional and district levels and service delivery personnel at health centers. These programs include: the Reproductive and Child Health Unit's programs focused on early childhood care, neonatal care, school health services, adolescent health services, antenatal care, and maternal health; and the Expanded Programme on Immunization; the National Malaria Control Programme; the National Tuberculosis and Leprosy Control Programme; and the National HIV/AIDS Control Programme.

As we hope this discussion shows, Tanzania has a healthcare system that is fairly well distributed. About 80 percent of the population has access to health services; over 90 percent lives within ten kilometers (six miles) of a healthcare facility of some form. The majority of the country's roughly 5,000 health facilities are located in rural areas, where 75 percent of the population resides.

Tanzania's Healthcare Workforce

Tanzania has had a long history of shortage in its health workforce. At the time of the mainland's independence in 1961, there were a mere 415 physicians in the entire country, only 12 of whom were Tanzanians.[13] Today, Tanzania has 1,339 doctors (884 in the public sector and 455 in the private sector) for its population of forty million people, a ratio of fewer than 3.4 physicians per 100,000 population. Fifty-two percent of doctors work in the Dar es Salaam region, which has a doctor-to-population ratio six times higher than the national average. Fourteen out of twenty-six regions in the country have fewer than one doctor per 100,000 people. Because of the scarcity of physicians, a range of other healthcare providers, such as assistant medical officers (AMOs), perform many of the functions of physicians. AMOs receive clinical training similar to that of general physicians. The total number of AMOs in Tanzania is about the same as physicians, and the majority (74 percent) work in the public sector. Clinical officers, another level of health personnel, have less clinical training than AMOs but are much more numerous than doctors or AMOs. There are 6,908 clinical officers (18 per 100,000 people) in Tanzania.[14]

Muhimbili University of Health and Allied Sciences (MUHAS), in Dar es Salaam, is the only government-supported school training doctors, nurses, dentists, and pharmacists. Currently, there are four private medical schools training doctors in the country: Hubert Kairuki Memorial University and Vignan's International Medical and Technological University, both in Dar es Salaam; Tumaini University, an affiliate of the Kilimanjaro Christian Medical College, in Kilimanjaro; and Bugando University College of Health Sciences, in Mwanza. Tanzania has approximately 105 nursing and allied health-training institutions. Of these, the government owns 70; the remaining 35 are owned by religious organizations.

Healthcare Financing and Health Insurance

Tanzania spends 1.7 percent of its GDP on health, an expenditure of $29 per person.[15] A mix of financing sources is used to support the health system. About 70 percent of the funding is from public financing through taxation, but patients share costs by paying user fees at government health facilities.

At present, general primary healthcare services are provided by the government free of charge to children up to age five and to pregnant women. Free care is also provided to patients with HIV/AIDS and tuberculosis (TB), under focused government programs. The remainder of the population can receive medical exams free of charge at public facilities but must pay for diagnostic tests and any treatments that are prescribed. A number of public and private insurance schemes are available to Tanzanians. However, the number of people covered remains very small.

Leading Health Issues in Tanzania

HIV/AIDS

Since the first three cases of HIV/AIDS were reported in Tanzania in 1983,[16] the HIV/AIDS epidemic has had a devastating effect on every sector of Tanzanian society. Gains in national economic growth during earlier decades were reversed by the untimely deaths of large numbers of people in their most economically productive years, and by the financial toll incurred from providing care to HIV-infected patients. At the peak of the epidemic in the late 1990s, up to 50 percent of hospital beds were occupied by patients with HIV/AIDS-related illnesses;[17] life expectancy reached an all-time low of fifty-one years in 2008. The country has experienced a rapid increase in the number of AIDS orphans as more and more children have lost one or both parents to the disease. Nearly every Tanzanian has been affected, directly or indirectly, by the epidemic. In response, Tanzania's government launched a comprehensive program to address the crisis. In December 1999, then-president Benjamin William Mkapa boldly declared the HIV/AIDS situation in Tanzania to be a national disaster and "called upon the entire nation" to undertake "new measures to put the nation on a war-footing against HIV/AIDS."[18] Such strong support from the highest level has ensured that responding to the HIV/AIDS epidemic remains a top priority for the government.

National efforts to prevent and control HIV/AIDS have been robust and far-reaching. Tanzania serves as an example of what can be achieved through vigorous government response coupled with international assistance. In 1985, two years after the first cases were diagnosed, the MOHSW launched an action plan to address HIV/AIDS and announced the formation of an AIDS Task Force, which later became the country's National AIDS Control Programme. The government released its National Policy on HIV/AIDS in 2001. That same year, an act of Parliament established the Tanzania Commission for AIDS under the prime minister's office to "facilitate and strengthen the expanded response to the epidemic."[19] The commission provides strategic leadership, guides implementation of the country's action plan for AIDS, and is responsible for coordinating, monitoring, and evaluating the national response to the epidemic. The U.S. Centers for Disease Control and Prevention (CDC) established a Global AIDS Program Tanzania Office in 2001. The CDC has worked closely with the National AIDS Control Programme to support outreach and prevention activities, develop national blood transfusion services and guidelines on the appropriate use of blood products, and provide technical assistance on HIV care and treatment priorities.[20] These intensive efforts have been effective at stemming, though not reversing, the epidemic. In 2007, HIV prevalence was estimated to be 6.2 percent,[21] with prevalence having remained constant in the Tanzanian mainland since 2001. Women have higher rates of HIV infection than men in Tanzania. This is probably due to a variety of factors, including issues of gender inequality and a higher likelihood of HIV transmission to the female partner during unprotected heterosexual intercourse.[22]

The introduction of antiretroviral medications on a mass scale has significantly increased the willingness of individuals to be tested for HIV and is slowly eroding the stigma associated with HIV/AIDS. A diagnosis of HIV infection is no longer considered a death sentence. Just as is now the case in the United States, in Tanzania, a diagnosis of HIV is viewed as a serious but treatable condition. Antiretroviral therapy (ART; see the glossary) first became available in Tanzania in 2002, but only to those who could afford it. The cost at that time was more than $1,000 per year, and it was estimated that fewer than 2,000 patients were on ART by the end of 2003. Over the ensuing years, HIV/AIDS care and treatment guidelines were published, and training of Tanzanian healthcare providers in the use and monitoring of these medicines began.

With support from several international entities such as the Global Fund to Fight AIDS, Tuberculosis and Malaria, the President's Emergency Plan For AIDS Relief (PEPFAR), and the Clinton Foundation (see the glossary for all three), the Tanzanian government established a network of HIV/AIDS care and treatment centers for adults and children throughout the country. These international and partner agencies have established regions throughout Tanzania in which each is responsible for the delivery of HIV diagnosis, care, and treatment services. There are now more than twenty centers throughout the country that offer same-day HIV testing using rapid diagnostic test kits, and free treatment services to adults and children. The rapid scale-up of ART programs has been remarkable. Of the roughly 1.6 million Tanzanians living with HIV in 2006, more than 568,800 were receiving care and support, and more than 83,300 were receiving ART. By mid-2008, the number of patients receiving ART had doubled to over 160,000.[23]

Heterosexual sex is the most common route of transmission for HIV in Tanzania, responsible for approximately 80 percent of infections. An estimated 18 percent of infections are due to mother-to-child-transmission, with less than 5 percent due to blood transfusions, intravenous drug use and needle-stick injuries, or traditional practices which involve cutting.[24] Overall, 6.2 percent of the population between the ages of fifteen and forty-nine is HIV-infected.[25] The epidemic is not evenly distributed in the country, however. Regions with the highest prevalence include Iringa (14.7 percent), Dar es Salaam (8.9 percent), Mbeya (7.9 percent), and Shinyanga (7.6 percent); regions with the lowest rates include Zanzibar (0.6 percent), Kigoma (0.9 percent), Arusha (1.4 percent), and Manyara (1.7 percent).[26]

Stigma and discrimination are pervasive and persistent barriers both to patients being tested for HIV and to their receiving care. Our experience has taught us that many patients are uncomfortable sharing their HIV status with their friends or families. In one of our clinical trials in the early 2000s, we asked HIV-positive participants to identify a person we could contact if they became ill. More than half of our participants reported they had not informed anyone of their HIV status. In our pediatric HIV program, HIV-infected mothers report being afraid to use formula to feed their infants, rather than breast-feed, for fear that their family members and their wider community will assume that they are HIV-infected and shun or ostracize them. Our patients routinely ask that we not make home visits so that they do not need to fabricate stories about why a nurse is visiting them or their children. Reducing this fear and stigma has been tackled through education campaigns challenging prevailing myths about HIV transmission through casual contact, and promoting the concept that HIV is a treatable disease.

Prevention of HIV transmission has been an important component of the country's comprehensive plan to address the epidemic. Programs to prevent mother-to-child transmission (PMTCT; see the glossary) of HIV were initially piloted at five sites in 2000. Today over 2,400 health facilities throughout the country that offer reproductive health services provide such programs, not as a separate, vertical HIV/AIDS program, but integrated into antenatal care services. All women enrolled in antenatal care are offered voluntary HIV testing. If a woman tests positive for HIV during pregnancy, she is enrolled in a program to prevent mother-to-child transmission. Current guidelines in Tanzania use the standard single dose of neviripine regimen: a dose of neviripine is given to the mother during labor, and then a single dose is given to the infant within seventy-two hours of delivery. This intervention cuts the risk of HIV transmission during labor and delivery in half, from roughly 25 percent to 30 percent down to 12 percent to 15 percent.[27] Single dose neviripine remains the regimen of choice in areas that are unable to initiate ART. Where ART is available, Tanzanian national guidelines recommend a multidrug regimen. Sometimes neviripine is part of the regimen, but the point is multidrug versus single drug regimen—that is, combining drugs with different mechanisms of action for pregnant women.[28] The use of multidrug ART (or combination therapy, as it is called, because it combines drugs with different mechanisms of action) is estimated to further reduce the transmission risk to 4 percent to 6 percent.[29]

HIV prevention efforts have also included social marketing campaigns and school-based education programs to inform youth about the risk of HIV and how to protect themselves from infection. The message of the main educational campaigns has followed the well-known "ABC" approach: Abstinence before marriage (also referred to as delaying sexual debut), Being monogamous in one's relationship, and using Condoms. Social marketing campaigns communicate educational and anti-stigma messages and encourage testing through songs, posters, rallies, and the media. To launch a national AIDS awareness campaign in 2007, President Jakaya Mrisho Kikwete and his wife publicly underwent HIV testing, along with several other high-level political officials.[30] This set an important example for the rest of the country. Ishi, the Kiswahili word for live, is an awareness and education program that focuses on behavior change among fifteen- to nineteen-year-olds. The multimedia Femina Health Information Project adds gender equality and civic education to its HIV prevention and sexual health messages. Overall, the government, FBOs, and NGOs have been very supportive of each other's campaigns.

The HIV/AIDS epidemic has markedly affected family structure, social expectations, education, and communities in Tanzania (see the sidebar on AIDS orphans). Eleven percent of the nation's children under eighteen have lost one or both parents to illness.[31] The distribution of orphaned children closely follows the distribution of the HIV/AIDS epidemic in the country.[32]

Tuberculosis

In 2009, Tanzania ranked fifteenth in the world in terms of burden of TB, based on the estimated annual number of new TB cases arising worldwide.[33] Similar to its response to the HIV/AIDS epidemic, the government has a vigorous national campaign to control TB. As a result, the incidence rate of new cases of TB decreased by more than 4 percent (from 312 to 297 cases per 100,000 population) between 2006 and 2007.[34] Tanzania's National Tuberculosis and Leprosy Programme (NTLP) was established in 1977, and in 2006, the president declared TB to be a national emergency.[35]

BEN ROBBINS AND BRIAN CHRISTIE

We decided to create SALAMA: Tanzania, a nonprofit organization, after a summer internship in Tanzania. SALAMA stands for Students for the Advancement of Learning and Medical Aid. In Swahili, it means peace or safety.

In the summer of 2007, we traveled to Mbagala, a poor neighborhood on the outskirts of Dar es Salaam, to work at the Bibi Jann School, a small, self-supported elementary school aimed at educating children living in the most extreme poverty of the surrounding area. There we taught basic English, science, and math to children in first, second, and third grades. Although the youngsters were incredibly bright and motivated, they suffered huge disadvantages because of the financial situation in their homes and their school. Many talked about wanting to become doctors or nurses, but without books, with recurring illnesses from numerous preventable causes, and with teachers chronically unpaid and on the verge of leaving, there weren't sufficient resources to prepare the students for secondary school.

We wanted to ensure that the children had the needed support to complete a high-quality primary education so that they could continue to secondary school, and their opportunities would not be limited. To understand how best to assist the students, we asked the school director to provide a list of the most pressing needs. Everything he wanted—chalk, desks, classroom space, additional teaching staff—could be addressed by fundraising among family and friends in the United States.

Upon returning to the United States, we started SALAMA: Tanzania with the idea that well-structured financial support could address many major concerns for the future of the children at the school. We started fundraising in our hometown communities and at our school, Dartmouth College. We completed an application to establish our organization as a 501(c)(3) nonprofit entity to support children's educational activities. We have raised over $80,000, which has been used to build classrooms, pay salaries, and purchase school supplies. Plans to support the school's relocation to a larger site and expand it through sixth grade are under way. Our short-term stay in Tanzania created a long-term commitment to ensure that the children at Bibi Jann's have the opportunity to pursue their goals.

BEN ROBBINS graduated from Dartmouth College in 2008 as a psychology major. He has been to Tanzania twice, first as a Dartmouth DarDar-Dickey Intern in summer 2007, and again as a Lombard Fellow during winter/spring 2010. He began attending Harvard Medical School in the fall of 2010.

BRIAN CHRISTIE is a Nashville native who graduated from Dartmouth College in 2007 as a creative writing major. After spending the 2007–8 school year in Tanzania as a Lombard Fellow, he entered Duke Medical School.

Tanzania has been referred to as the "birthplace of the DOTS strategy" (see the glossary), which is the internationally accepted strategy for controlling TB. It was in Tanzania that Dr. Karel Styblo, working in collaboration with local authorities, developed and implemented this novel approach to TB control in the 1970s. With its network of DOTS clinics throughout the country, the NTLP is responsible for diagnosing and treating all patients with TB. When treatment is initiated, patients are assigned a NTLP number and given a TB card (often referred to as the "green card"), which is a mini-medical record summarizing the status of the patient's treatment course. The standard of care for TB in Tanzania and throughout the world is to provide treatment using directly observed therapy. This requires that a trained healthcare worker (such as a nurse, physician, or trained community health worker) observes and documents patients taking their medications. Treatment is done primarily on an outpatient basis; only the most ill patients who may also need intravenous medicines or fluids are hospitalized.

As evidence of the government's commitment to controlling TB in Tanzania, anti-tuberculosis medicines are distributed free of charge to all collaborating service providers, including NGOs and private for-profit health facilities. State-of-the-art TB treatment uses fixed-dose-combination tablets to improve patient adherence and reduce prescribing errors; these tablets were recently introduced in priority areas of the country. As in most countries, anti-tuberculosis medications are tightly regulated by the government and dispensed only at government-approved clinics. This is done primarily to prevent misuse of these drugs, which can lead to the emergence of drug-resistant organisms.

There is very little drug-resistant TB in Tanzania; only 1.1 percent of new TB cases in 2007 were multidrug-resistant TB (MDR TB; see the glossary).[36] However in 2006, as drug-resistant strains increased worldwide, the NTLP developed plans and protocols for managing MDR TB, including the construction of appropriate hospital wards and laboratories to conduct drug-susceptibility testing. Full-scale management of MDR TB began the following year.

In response to the overlapping epidemics of TB and HIV/AIDS, the NTLP began collaborative TB-HIV activities in seventy districts in 2007, to address the complicated care and treatment issues of coinfection. World Health Organization (WHO; see the glossary) guidelines recommend that all patients diagnosed with TB be routinely tested for HIV (patients may refuse testing), and all patients diagnosed with HIV infection be evaluated for TB. This practice is the standard of care in Tanzania's HIV and TB clinics, along with providing co-trimoxazole (to prevent certain opportunistic infections) to HIV-infected TB patients and offering ART at TB clinics for increasingly coordinated care.[37]

Malaria

Tanzania is among the 31 countries with the highest burden of malaria cases.[38] Malaria poses a serious threat in Tanzania; in 2007 there were more than 10 million cases of malaria which resulted in more than 12,000 deaths, mostly in children under five, the most vulnerable age group. In a recent national household survey, the overall prevalence of malaria in young children was 18 percent. Prevalence increased by age in children under five, from 9 percent in infants ages six to eleven months to 22 percent among children forty-eight to fifty-nine months. Malaria prevalence in children is not evenly distributed throughout the country: it was highest in the Kagera region (42 percent in children under five) and lowest in Arusha (1 percent). Other regions with high prevalence rates (30 percent or more) include Lindi, Mara, Mtwara, Mwanza, and Shinyanga.[39]

Tanzania's National Malaria Control Programme oversees diagnostic, treatment, and preventive services related to malaria. Tests have revealed high levels of resistance to first-line antimalarial drugs such as chloroquine and sulphadoxine-pyrimethamine (Fansidar). Consequently, Tanzania's 2006 national Malaria Guidelines recommend the use of artemisinin-based combination therapy.[40] Artermeter-Lumefantrin (ALU) is the preferred treatment for uncomplicated malaria. At present, resistance to artemisinin-based combination therapy has not been documented in Tanzania. Due to a shortage of laboratory facilities for diagnosing malaria and the high mortality among young children, it is the national policy to presumptively treat children under age five for malaria based on clinical symptoms. However, the malaria program has recognized the potential for overtreatment of malaria (and consequently the mistreatment of febrile illnesses due to other causes) and is shifting from a clinically based diagnostic approach to one based on laboratory testing.

Malaria prevention is also a national priority. Efforts are focused on distributing insecticide-treated bed nets and indoor residual spraying (see below). Most bed nets used in Tanzania have been treated with pyrethroids, which have low mammalian toxicity, serve as both a repellent and a toxic agent to mosquitoes, and are odorless and stable over long periods. In 2007–8, thirty-nine percent of households reported owning at least one net, up from 23 percent in 2004–5. Approximately 26 percent of children under five and pregnant women had slept under a net the night before the survey. Urban dwellers are much more likely (in some cases twice as likely) to own and to have their children under five and pregnant women sleep under a net than their rural counterparts. The government program has set as targets that 90 percent of households will own at least one treated net, and 85 percent of pregnant women and children under five will sleep under nets by 2012.[41]

Vector control through indoor residual spraying—the scheduled spraying of an insecticide on the inside walls of homes—is another core prevention activity. The spraying interrupts malaria transmission by killing the female mosquito when she enters a home and rests on the wall. In Tanzania, spraying began in 2001 in just one district and has been expanded widely since then, with a goal of reaching 38 of the 120 districts between 2008 and 2012.[42] In addition, the use of microbial larvicides—placing larvicidal agents in standing water where mosquitoes breed — has been reintroduced in the past few years in specified research areas, with planned future expansion.

Issues in Child Health

Nearly 188,000 Tanzanian children under five die each year. Approximately 90 percent of all childhood deaths are attributable to common and preventable illnesses such as malaria, pneumonia, diarrhea, malnutrition, and HIV/AIDS-related complications of low birth weight.[43] Tanzania has an astoundingly high infant mortality rate, with nearly 70 infants per 1,000 live births dying before their first birthday, and 118 children per 1,000 live births dying before age five.

Almost 80 percent of healthcare facilities in the country offer basic child health services, including outpatient treatment, childhood immunizations, and growth monitoring. The availability of children's health services varies across the country: childhood immunization services are least available in facilities in the eastern zone and Zanzibar, and more available in the central and southern zones.

Tanzania is implementing the Integrated Management of Childhood Illness, IMCI, strategy (see the glossary). Tanzania has included IMCI in its national package of essential health interventions, a major component of the national health policy. Since the introduction of IMCI, the quality of care for sick children has improved, leading to a 13 percent reduction in child mortality and a significant reduction in poor growth indicators such as stunting.[44] IMCI costs less annually per child ($4) than routine care ($26).

The MOHSW's Expanded Programme on Immunization aims to ensure that all children are fully immunized by their first birthday. All basic program vaccines for the seven major childhood diseases[45] are available in three-fourths of eligible facilities. Sixty-two percent of children under twelve months and 71 percent of children twelve to twenty-three months are fully vaccinated.[46]

Breast-feeding and Nutritional Status

Breast-feeding by a healthy mother is universally endorsed by medical experts as the best way to feed infants, as it supports optimal child development and protects against acute and chronic illnesses. Almost all children in Tanzania are breast-fed, with 41 percent being exclusively breast-fed for at least six months. The majority of children (91 percent) receive supplemental foods in addition to breast-feeding between six and nine months, and 55 percent still breast-feed at twenty to thirty months of age.[47]

There are some specific challenges to breast-feeding in settings such as Tanzania. HIV can be transmitted to a child from an HIV-infected mother via breast milk. The need to mix formula with clean water, which may not be readily available in all settings, further complicates the choice to breast-feed or use formula. Currently, WHO recommends HIV-infected mothers exclusively breast-feed their children for the first six months of life unless replacement feeding is acceptable, feasible, affordable, sustainable, and safe for them and their infants.[48] Tanzania's MOHSW has adopted this policy as well.

Protein-energy malnutrition is the most widespread and leading nutritional disorder in Tanzania, most commonly affecting children ages six months to five years. The condition results from lack of food or from infections that cause loss of appetite while increasing the body's nutrient requirements and losses. Nationally 44 percent of children younger than five are stunted (under the normal height for their age), 17 percent are underweight, 3 percent are wasted, and 22 percent have both chronic and acute undernutrition. The prevalence of stunting is far higher among rural children than urban children. Only 4 percent of Tanzanian children under five are overweight.[49]

Agencies, Initiatives, and Other Partners in Tanzania

Working in Tanzania will introduce you to a wide range of agencies and health initiatives. We have highlighted a few of the key organizations here to give you a flavor of the numerous international and interagency collaborations.

WHO opened a Country Office in Tanzania in 1963 to support the country's national health authorities. The office "also coordinates and builds partnerships with sister UN agencies, other multilateral and bilateral agencies, learning and research institutions, civil societies (NGOs and CBOs) and professional associations."[50]

Since 1989, the African Medical and Research Foundation, Tanzania, together with the MOHSW, has been implementing a range of HIV-prevention activities among truck drivers (a known high-risk group for HIV infection). Its pilot project, involving two major trucking companies and seven truck stops along a major trucking route, has been expanded nationally.

The CDC's office in Dar es Salaam plays a critical role in healthcare program development, training, and infrastructure development in Tanzania. In addition to being one of the lead U.S. governmental management agencies for PEPFAR, the CDC supports Tanzania's National Malaria Control Programme as part of the President's Malaria Initiative (PMI; see the glossary). Since 2005, this effort has produced marked gains in access to malaria prevention and treatment interventions through the provision of insecticide-treated bed nets, indoor residual spraying, intermittent treatment for pregnant women, and access to artemisinin-based combination therapies.

The CDC's Global AIDS Program has worked with the MOHSW since February 2001, to support outreach activities targeting the most at-risk populations, prevention of mother-to-child HIV transmission, development of national blood transfusion services, guidelines on the appropriate use of blood products, technical assistance for integration of HIV and TB services, and voluntary HIV counseling and testing. The program collaborates with the Tanzanian government and its other partners to strengthen laboratory infrastructure and capacity for HIV diagnosis, staging of disease severity based on WHO criteria, and therapeutic monitoring, as well as strengthening capacity around TB and HIV issues.

Former U.S. President Bill Clinton established the Clinton HIV/AIDS Initiative in 2002. As part of the Clinton Foundation's Global Initiative, this program works with governments to improve ART access and the healthcare systems required to deliver these crucial medicines. The foundation's work in Tanzania includes extensive program development with several national ministries on HIV prevention and testing, guidelines development, and antiretroviral medication procurement, specifically low-cost generics.

Tanzania was one of PEPFAR's original focus countries; it began supporting HIV/AIDS activities in Tanzania in 2004, with an allocation of over $70 million that year. The amount of support has grown each year; in fiscal year 2008, PEPFAR provided $313.4 million to Tanzania. PEPFAR funds are distributed through more than a hundred primary partners and subpartners, which include national, regional, and international NGOS, FBOS, and academic institutions. In Tanzania, PEPFAR funds are managed through five U.S. agencies: the Department of Defense, the CDC (which is part of the Department of Health and Human Services), the Peace Corps, the Department of State, and the U.S. Agency for International Development (USAID; see the glossary).

Numerous international NGOS are active in Tanzania. Several websites offering comprehensive guides to NGOS provide more specific information.[51] You may be familiar with some of the more prominent groups currently working in Tanzania, including Doctors Without Borders, WaterAid America, Direct Relief International, and Project Concern International.[52]

In addition, there are about 1,500 national or local NGOS operating in Tanzania. Most of these operate at the regional or district level, and collectively they offer a wide range of support in all areas of development in Tanzania. Their activities are coordinated by the Tanzania Association of NGOS, known as TANGO. Of local NGOS, more than 100 support HIV/AIDS activities in mainland Tanzania with activities that include research, consultancy, counseling, behavior change, income generation, capacity building, advocacy, education, family planning, home-based care, and orphan care.

Many universities throughout the world are establishing partnerships with the Tanzanian government and with the major universities and teaching hospitals in the country. In addition to our Dartmouth partnership[53] with Muhimbili University of Health and Allied Sciences (MUHAS), in Dar es Salaam, other universities with partnerships in the country include the Global Health Science Program of the University of California, San Francisco; Harvard School of Public Health's Global Research Program; the Karolinska Institute of Stockholm; and Columbia University's Mailman School of Public Health.[54]

The Dartmouth and Dar es Salaam (DarDar) Programs: A Multifaceted Partnership

Dartmouth's Global Health Initiative is a program of Dartmouth Medical School and the College's Dickey Center for International Understanding. Tanzania was selected as a site for the initiative's activities because two previously established programs had fostered a broad-based collaborative relationship between Dartmouth and MUHAS. Both institutions signed a memorandum of understanding in 2005, solidifying their commitment to undertake joint, sustainable, and replicable programs to address global health priorities by leveraging the strengths of each institution. Programs provide interdisciplinary educational and research opportunities for students, faculty, and researchers at both institutions. The MUHAS-Dartmouth collaboration perfectly exemplifies the hoped-for partnerships and linkages anticipated by the Global Health Initiative, as the programs described below demonstrate.

The DarDar (Dartmouth-Dar es Salaam) Health Study, a clinical trial of a TB vaccine in HIV-infected adults, was Dartmouth's first major research program in Tanzania. This Phase 3 randomized clinical trial assessed the efficacy of an inactivated mycobacterial vaccine booster to prevent HIV-associated TB. A clinical facility was constructed in Dar es Salaam, on-site vaccine immunology and TB laboratories were established, and detailed study protocols were developed and approved by institutional review boards at the participating institutions and government regulatory bodies. Between 2001 and 2008, over 4,000 patients were screened to identify 2,000 eligible HIV-infected participants who were randomized to receive either a five-dose series of the vaccine or a placebo over twelve months. Subjects were monitored regularly to detect new pulmonary TB or disseminated TB. The study found the vaccine to be safe and to provide significant protection against confirmed pulmonary TB in HIV-infected adults.[55] The DarDar site also offers training and internship opportunities for Dartmouth postgraduates, medical students, and undergraduates.

The Dartmouth-Boston University AIDS International Training and Research Program has had a wide-ranging impact since its establishment in 2003 on both the development of HIV research capacity at MUHAS and the national AIDS and TB policies in Tanzania. The program trains Tanzanian physician faculty in advanced molecular biology, epidemiology, public health, and clinical sciences applicable to HIV and provides short-term training focused on HIV or HIV-associated TB to Tanzanian physicians, researchers, library directors, and laboratory technologists. In addition, numerous in-country courses have been held including "TB in the Era of HIV," "Research Ethics in the Era of HIV," "Dermatology in the Era of HIV," "Reducing Mortality from HIV-associated TB," and "Nurses at the Forefront of HIV Care."

The DarDar Pediatric Program (DPP) was made possible by a grant from the Foundation for the Treatment of Children with AIDS in 2004. A joint venture between MUHAS and Dartmouth, the DPP provides care and treatment to infants, children, and adolescents with infected with HIV. It now receives additional support from the PEPFAR program in Tanzania. The DPP features a unique concept for Tanzania and most resource-limited countries — a clinic and staff dedicated exclusively to pediatric and adolescent HIV care. The DPP has already become a model for pediatric training and education in the greater Dar es Salaam region, and we are exploring the potential for DPP to serve as a pediatric HIV and TB educational resource for the entire country. Clinical research has focused on improving the diagnosis of TB latent infection and active disease in children. The DPP provides numerous training and research opportunities for undergraduate and graduate student interns from both Tanzania and the United States.

Reflections on Our Experience

As participants in the DarDar Programs for the past ten years, we have enjoyed a successful and productive collaboration in Tanzania, learning and growing together with our Tanzanian colleagues. If you are considering working in Tanzania, we offer two important insights.

First, we believe a critical component of our successful collaboration has been the concerted and intentional fostering of a truly balanced and equitable partnership. Throughout our endeavors, all major strategic decisions have been made with the involvement of the highest level of leadership at both institutions. All research and educational activities are undertaken jointly. This means that all of our major research endeavors include principal investigators from both institutions. Our student exchange programs are bilateral, with each institution both hosting and sending students.

Our second insight is that regular, scheduled, and ongoing communication is key. Collaborators from both sites participate in weekly conference calls to discuss the daily operations of projects, anticipate critical issues, and solve problems. All Tanzania-based directors and staff of the programs are Tanzanian. We constantly reevaluate our activities, realigning them as necessary to maintain the best balance. We place special emphasis on offering consistent, ongoing support and capacity-building for our junior collaborators in both countries. We believe that we have achieved the kind of balanced partnership that is so often desired in global health programs.

Conclusion

Tanzania is widely known for being receptive and welcoming to foreigners, and the two non-Tanzanian authors of this chapter can attest to the truth of that generalization. We have found our Tanzanian colleagues to be very warm, and we have enjoyed the friendships that have emerged from our professional relationships. Dar es Salaam is a hectic, dusty, bustling city, but one in which visitors can feel safe to explore (applying the usual street smarts that you need in any big urban center). It is not uncommon to hear people calling out *mzungu* to you as you walk around marketplaces or in villages where foreigners are less common. *Mzungu* is the Kiswahili word commonly used for any obvious foreigner, regardless of race, derived originally from a contraction of words meaning "one who moves around." While unsettling at first, this call is meant to catch your attention (perhaps to attract you to a vendor's stall); it is based on curiosity and is not meant to offend or intimidate you.

We instruct our students and other visitors to be conscious of and show respect for the social hierarchy established in all Tanzanian settings. A stricter professional hierarchy often means U.S. medical students experience a harsher grilling about the possible diagnoses and planned work-ups of their patients on the clinical wards than they are used to at home. We encourage students to welcome this careful probing of their knowledge.

Many of our students have described visits to busy marketplaces or a ride on one of the crowded mini vans (*dala dalas*) as an experience that represents their assimilation into life in Dar es Salaam. The *dala dalas* are the public bus system in Dar es Salaam and many travelers become quite adept at riding them (while constantly assessing their safety). Students have described the bus pulling up to the stop, doors wide open, people packed in as tightly as possible, women in their brightly colored *kangas* (wrap dresses), wind and red dust blowing around, and at every stop the driver starting up again before the money collector has gotten back on so that person has to run to catch up and hop on again. This is a common scene played over and over every day in Dar es Salaam. When travelers stop being startled at this sight, they know they have settled into their new surroundings.

Tanzania's health sector is complex, with many international and national partners contributing to its mission to provide comprehensive care to its citizens and address the burdens of disease. With its relative political stability, periods of economic growth, and dynamic health programs, Tanzania is poised to lead the way in progressive health efforts for many of its fellow African countries. The opportunity to work on a global health program in Tanzania, especially if through a well-established partnership or local organization, will promise an invaluable experience in a welcoming environment.

COUNTRY DATA : TANZANIA

Millennium Development Goal indicators are italicized.

TABLE 8.1 : **POPULATION AND HUMAN DEVELOPMENT**

POPULATION	
Total	40.2 million
Population growth rate	2.04%
Net migration rate/1,000 population	−1.43
Urban	25%
Rural	75%
AGE STRUCTURE	
0–14 years	43%
15–64 years	54.1%
65+ years	2.9%
Median age (years)	18
MAJOR ETHNIC GROUPS	
African (95% Bantu)	99%
Mainland: other (Asian, European, Arab)	1%
Zanzibar: Arab, African, mixed	NA
RELIGIONS	
Mainland: Christian	30%
Mainland: Muslim	35%
Mainland: indigenous	35%
Zanzibar: Muslim	> 99%
Zanzibar: other	< 1%
HUMAN DEVELOPMENT	
Human Development Index	0.503
Human Development rank[a]	152nd
Freedom House Index	Partly free
Political Rights score[b]	4
Civil Liberties score[b]	3
Human Poverty Index	32.5%
Human Poverty rank[c]	159th

Notes: [a]out of 179 countries; [b]1 = most free, 7 = least free; [c]out of 177 countries.

TABLE 8.2 : **GOVERNMENT AND ECONOMY**

GOVERNMENT	
Independence	Tanganyika: 9 Dec. 1961, from UK-administered UN trusteeship; Zanzibar: 19 Dec. 1963, from UK
Independent union formed	26 Apr. 1964
Type of government	Republic
Voting rights	Age 18, universal
CAPITAL	Dar es Salaam
CURRENCY	Tanzanian shilling (TZS)
ECONOMY	
Gross domestic product (GDP) (in PPP US $)	54.26 billion
Annual GDP growth	7.1%
GDP per capita (in US $)	$1,300
Gini Index	34.6
Population living below PPP $1/day	57.8%
External debt service as % of GDP	1.1
Public debt as % of GDP	22
Official development assistance (ODA) per capita (in US $)	$39.3
Foreign direct investment as % of GDP	3.9
LABOR FORCE	
In agriculture	80%
In industry and services, combined	20%
Unemployment rate	NA

TABLE 8.3 : **GEOGRAPHY AND ENVIRONMENT**

LAND COMPOSITION

Land area	945,087 sq. km. (364,900 sq. mi.), including islands of Mafia, Pemba, Zanzibar
Size comparison	Slightly larger than 2 x California
Terrain	Coastal plains, central plateau, highlands in north and south, 1,424-km. (884-mi.) coastline
Ecological hazards	Flooding on central plateau in rainy season, drought

LAND USE AND RESOURCES

Permanent crop land	1.2%
Arable land	4.2%
Agricultural products	Coffee, sisal, tea, cotton, pyrethrum, cashews, tobacco, corn, wheat, cassava, fruits, vegetables, livestock
Natural resources	Platinum, gemstones, gold, natural gas, hydropower, tin, phosphate, iron ore, coal, diamonds, nickel

ENVIRONMENTAL ISSUES   Soil degradation; deforestation; desertification; coral reef destruction threatens marine habitats; droughts affect marginal agriculture; wildlife threatened by illegal hunting

INFRASTRUCTURE

Population with access to improved water source	*45%*
Population using improved sanitation	*47%*
Roadways unpaved	91.4%

TABLE 8.4 : **HEALTH**

LIFE, BIRTH, DEATH

Life expectancy at birth (male/female)	50.5/53.5
Birth rate/1,000 population	34.29
Death rate/1,000 population	12.59
Infant mortality rate/1,000 live births	*69.28*

Physicians/100,000 population   3.4
Hospital beds/10,000 population   11

HEALTH ECONOMICS

Total expenditure on health per capita $29
   (PPP US $)
Public expenditure on health as % of GDP   1.7

DISEASES

Most common vector-borne diseases   Malaria, plague
Most common food- and water-borne diseases   Bacterial diarrhea,
                                                                   hepatitis A,
                                                                   typhoid fever,
                                                                   schistomosomiasis

TB incidence/100,000 population   *297*
TB prevalence/100,000 population   *459*
New TB cases HIV-positive   18%
New TB cases multidrug-resistant (MDR)   1.1%
TB deaths/100,000 population   66
Reported malaria cases annually   > 10 million
Malaria death rate/100,000 population   0.99
HIV prevalence rate in adults   *6.2%*
AIDS deaths in adults annually   *96,000*
People living with HIV   1.4 million
AIDS orphans   970,000

MATERNAL HEALTH

Fertility rate (children born per woman)   4.46
Contraceptive prevalence rate   *26%*
   (married women 15–49)
Maternal mortality rate/100,000 births   *950*
Lifetime risk of maternal death, 1 in: *24*
Births attended by skilled birth attendant   *43%*

CHILD HEALTH

Mortality rate of children < 5/1,000 live births   *118*
1-year-olds immunized against measles   *93%*
Children < 5 using insecticide-treated bed nets   *16%*
Children < 5 with fever treated   *58%*
   with antimalarial drugs
Newborns protected against tetanus   89%

HUNGER AND MALNUTRITION

Children < 5 underweight for age   *22%*
Children < 5 under height for age   *44%*
Population undernourished   *44%*

TABLE 8.5 : LANGUAGE, EDUCATION, AND LITERACY

LANGUAGES

Kiswahili	Official
English	Offical; primary language of commerce, administration, higher education
Arabic	
many local languages	

LITERACY

Adult literacy rate (population age 15+ who can read and write)	69.4%

EXPENDITURE

Public expenditure on education as % of GDP	2.2

EDUCATION

Primary mandatory	Yes
Secondary mandatory	Yes
Net enrollment in primary education[d]	98.0%
School life expectancy, in years (both genders)[e]	5.1

[d]Net enrollment rate in primary education is measured as the number of children of official primary school age who are enrolled in primary education as a percentage of children in the official primary school age population.

[e]School life expectancy is the total number of years of school (from primary through tertiary education) that a child can expect to receive.

Principal Sources for Data in Appendix Tables 8.1–8.5

Central Intelligence Agency, *The World Factbook* (https://www.cia.gov/library/publications/the-world-factbook/).

UNDP Human Development Report, 2007/2008, available at: www.hdrstats.undp.org.

UN Millennium Development Goals Indicators Database, available at: www.mdgs.un.org.

UNICEF. The State of the World's Children 2009. Available at: http://www.data.un.org.

WHO. Global Tuberculosis Control. Country Profile: United Republic of Tanzania. WHO Report 2008.

NOTES

1. Catie Lott and Bob Smith, editors, *Spectrum Guide to Tanzania*, 2nd American ed., Brooklyn, N.Y.: Interlink, 2002.

2. Central Intelligence Agency, The World Factbook. Tanzania. (https://www

.cia.gov/library/publications/the-world-factbook/geos/tz.html); United Republic of Tanzania, "Country Profile" (http://www.tanzania.go.tz/profilef.html).

3. United Republic of Tanzania, "Country Profile."

4. Catie Lott and Bob Smith, *Spectrum Guide to Tanzania.*

5. Chapter 1 gives an overview of the process of structural adjustment and the effects that ensued for many African countries.

6. Catie Lott and Bob Smith, *Spectrum Guide to Tanzania.*

7. United Republic of Tanzania, "Country Profile"; U.S. Committee for Refugees and Immigrants, "World Refugee Survey 2009" (http://www.refugees.org/countryreports.aspx?id=2346).

8. U.S. Department of State, International Religious Freedom Report 2007: Tanzania, Sept. 2007 (http://www.state.gov/g/drl/rls/irf/2007/90124.htm).

9. United Republic of Tanzania, "Country Profile"; *Spectrum Guide to Tanzania*; U.S. Department of State, Bureau of Democracy, Human Rights, and Labor (http://www.state.gov/g/drl/rls/hrrpt/2007/102128.htm).

10. "Reaching Africa's Highest Peaks: Tanzania," Advertising Supplement to the Wall Street Journal, produced and sponsored by Panorama Reports Ltd., 12 July 2008 (http://www.panoramareports-ltd.com/pdf/tanzania.pdf).

11. The United Republic of Tanzania, Ministry of Health, National Health Policy. February 1990. (http://www.tanzania.go.tz/pdf/Nationahealthpolicy .pdf).

12. Anders Arvidson and Mattias Norstrom, "Health Sector Policy Overview Paper," ENABLE project, whose full title is "Building capacity in renewables in the health, education and water sectors to help meet poverty reduction targets in sub-Saharan Africa," September 2006 (http://www.enable.nu/publication/D_1_7_Tanzania_Health_Policy_Overview.pdf).

13. Anitta Juntunen, "Professional and Lay Care in the Tanzanian Village of Ilembula," academic dissertation, Faculty of Medicine, University of Oulu, Oulu, Finland, 2001 (http://herkules.oulu.fi/isbn9514264312/html/x325.html), chapter 3.

14. National Bureau of Statistics (NBS) [Tanzania] and Macro International Inc., Tanzania Service Provision Assessment Survey 2006, Dar es Salaam, Tanzania: National Bureau of Statistics and Macro International Inc, 2007 (http://www.measuredhs.com/pubs/pdf/SPA12/SPA12.pdf).

15. United Nations Development Programme, Human Development Report 2007/2008 (http://hdr.undp.org/en/media/HDR_20072008_EN_complete.pdf)

16. Tanzania Commission for AIDS, "National Multi-Sectoral Strategic Framework on HIV/AIDS, 2003–2007" Dar es Salaam, Tanzania: Prime Minister's Office, January 2003.

17. Tanzania National AIDS Control Programme, "AIDS in Africa during the Nineties" Dar es Salaam, Tanzania: Tanzania National Bureau of Statistics, 2001.

18. Benjamin William Mkapa, "New Year Message to the Nation," Dar es Salaam, Tanzania, 31 December 1999. National Multi-Sectoral Strategic Framework on HIV/AIDS, 2003–2007.

19. Central Intelligence Agency, The World Factbook. Tanzania.

20. Centers for Disease Control and Prevention, "Global HIV/AIDS Activities Tanzania" (http://www.cdc.gov/globalaids/Global-HIV-AIDS-at-CDC/countries/Tanzania/).

21. Tanzania Commission for AIDS, "UNGASS Country Progress Report: Tanzania Mainland" (30 January 2008; http://data.unaids.org/pub/Report/2008/tanzania_2008_country_progress_report_en.pdf).

22. UNAIDS, "Increase Women's Control over HIV Prevention—Fight AIDS: Global Coalition on Women and AIDS," Issue Brief #4 (2005; http://data.unaids.org/pub/BriefingNote/2006/20060530_FS_women%27s%20HIV%20Prevention%20Control_en.pdf).

23. Tanzanian Ministry of Health and Social Welfare, "National Guidelines for the Management of HIV/AIDS" (2008; http://www.moh.go.tz/documents/Tanzania_national_guidelines_2009.pdf).

24. Tanzania Commission for HIV/AIDS, "The Second Multi-Sectoral Strategic Framework on HIV/AIDS 2008–2012" Dar es Salaam, Tanzania: Prime Minister's Office, (October 2007; http://www.tacaids.go.tz/documents/NMSF%20%202008%20-2012.pdf).

25. Tanzania HIV/AIDS and Malaria Indicator Survey 2007–08, Preliminary Report, National Bureau of Statistics, Tanzania, (July 2008; http://www.ihi.or.tz/docs/TzHIV-MalariaIndicatorSurvey-07-08-PreliminaryReport.pdf).

26. Ibid.

27. L. A. Guay et al., "Intrapartum and Neonatal Single-dose Nevirapine Compared with Zidovudine for Prevention of Mother-to-child Transmission of HIV-1 in Kampala, Uganda: HIVNET 012 Randomised Trial," Lancet 354, no. 9181 (1999): 795–802.

28. Tanzania, Ministry of Health and Social Welfare, "National Guidelines for the Prevention of Mother to Child Transmission of HIV" (2007; http://www.aidstar-one.com/sites/default/files/treatment_documents/hiv_treatment_guidelines_tanzania_pmtct_2005.pdf).

29. World Health Organization, WHO Statistical Information System (WHOSIS), "HIV-infected Pregnant Women Receiving Antiretroviral Therapy for PMTCT (percentage)" (http://www.who.int/whosis/indicators/compendium/2008/2pmf/en/index.html).

30. PEPFAR. "Stories of Hope. Tanzania Launches National HIV/AIDS Testing Campaign," (September 2007; http://www.pepfar.gov/press/92135.htm).

31. Tanzania HIV/AIDS and Malaria Indicator Survey 2007–08.

32. Tanzania 2007. In Iringa, where the HIV prevalence is highest in the

country, 23.6 percent of children have lost one or both parents; in regions such as Mara, where HIV prevalence is lower than the national average, 14.7 percent of children are single or double orphans.

33. WHO, "Global Tuberculosis Control: Epidemiology, Strategy, Financing," WHO Report 2009. Geneva: World Health Organization (WHO/HTM/TB/2009 .411); (http://www.who.int/tb/publications/global_report/2009/en/index .html).

34. Ibid.

35. Ibid.

36. Ibid.

37. Ibid.

38. World Health Organization, "World Malaria Report 2009" Geneva: World Health Organization, (2009; http://whqlibdoc.who.int/publications/2009/ 9789241563901_eng.pdf).

39. Tanzania HIV/AIDS and Malaria Indicator Survey 2007-08.

40. Tanzania Ministry of Health, National Malaria Control Programme, "Malaria Guidelines," Dar es Salaam, Tanzania, 2006.

41. Tanzania proposal to the Global Fund to Fight AIDS, Tuberculosis and Malaria, round 7, Submitted July 2007 (http://www.theglobalfund.org/ grantdocuments/7TNZM_1589_0_full.pdf).

42. Ibid.

43. World Health Organization, WHO Statistical Information System (WHOSIS), "Mortality Country Fact Sheet 2006: United Republic of Tanzania" (http://www.who.int/whosis/mort/profiles/mort_afro_tza_tanzania.pdf).

44. J. R. Armstrong Schellenberg et al., "Effectiveness and Cost of Facility-based Integrated Management of Childhood Illness (IMCI) in Tanzania," *Lancet* 364, no. 9445 (2004): 1583-94.

45. The vaccines in the program include BCG (for TB), polio, diphtheria, pertusis, tetanus, and measles, and HIB (for *Hemophilus influenzae* type b, the most common cause of meningitis in childhood).

46. Tanzania, National Bureau of Statistics, and Macro International Inc, "Tanzania Demographic and Health Survey 2004-05" (Dar es Salaam: National Bureau of Statistics and ORC Macro, 2005). Survey report can be downloaded as separate chapters at http://www.measuredhs.com/pubs/pub_details.cfm?ID= 566&ctry_id=39&SrchTp=ctry#dfiles.

47. World Health Organization, "World Health Statistics 2007," Geneva: WHO (2007; http://www.who.int/whosis/whostat2007.pdf).

48. World Health Organization, "Child and Adolescent Health and Development: HIV and Infant Feeding" (http://www.who.int/child_adolescent_health/ topics/prevention_care/child/nutrition/hivif/en/index.html).

49. World Health Organization, "World Health Statistics 2007."

50. World Health Organization, "WHO in Tanzania" (http://www.who.int/countries/tza/who_in_tanzania/en/).

51. Guides to NGOs worldwide are available at the following website (http://www.wango.org/resources.aspx?section=ngodir&sub=region&regionID=30&col=f85038) and NonProfitExpert.com, "Tanzania." (http://www.nonprofitexpert.com/countries/tanzania.htm).

52. Doctors without Borders is also known as Médecins sans Frontières (http://www.doctorswithoutborders.org/news/country.cfm?id=2371); WaterAid America, "Tanzania." (http://www.wateraidamerica.org/what_we_do/where_we_work/tanzania/default.aspx?gclid=COKokvjvk5gCFQt4Hgod2Avsng); Direct Relief International, "Tanzania" (http://www.directrelief.org/WhereWeWork/Countries/Tanzania/Tanzania.aspx); Project Concern International, "Tanzania." (http://www.projectconcern.org/site/PageServer?pagename=Providing_clean_water_and_improving_family_health_in_Tanzania).

53. http://dickey.dartmouth.edu/initiatives/ghi.

54. Global Health Science Program of the University of California, San Francisco (http://www.globalhealthsciences.ucsf.edu/programs/muhas-partnership/index.aspx); Harvard School of Public Health, Global Research, "Tanzania" (https://webapps.sph.harvard.edu/cfdocs/worldmap/view.cfm?country=tanzania); Karolinska Institute (http://ki.se/ki/jsp/polopoly.jsp?d=36026&l=en); Columbia University, International Center for AIDS Care and Treatment Programs, "Tanzania" (http://www.columbia-icap.org/wherewework/tanzania/).

55. Charles F. von Reyn et al., "Prevention of Tuberculosis in Bacille Calmette-Guérin-primed, HIV-infected Adults Boosted with an Inactivated Whole-cell Mycobacterial Vaccine," *AIDS* 24, no. 5 (2010): 675-85.

SUGGESTED READING AND VIEWING

Film

David Breashears. *Kilimanjaro: To the Roof of Africa*. Washington, D.C., National Geographic, 2002.

Anne Macksoud and John Ankele, directors/filmmakers. *Grandmother to Grandmother: New York to Tanzania*. Woodstock, Vt., Old Dog Documentaries, 2009. (This film introduces two outstanding projects—one in the Bronx, N.Y., one in Tanzania—that are finding simple and effective ways to support grandmothers who are raising grandchildren orphaned by AIDS and other causes. The film can be obtained from http://olddogdocumentaries.com/.)

Hubert Sauper. *Darwin's Nightmare*. Paris, France, Celluloid Dreams, 2004. (This award-winning 2004 French-Belgian-Austrian documentary addresses the environmental and social effects of the fishing industry around Lake

Victoria in Tanzania. This film attracted criticism from the fisheries in the country and from the Tanzanian President Jakaya Kikwete who set up a special parliamentary committee to investigate the film's effect on the fishing industry. The controversy sparked by this film, based on whether its portrayal of the industry and local inhabitants was accurate and/or damaging, remains with advocates on both sides.

Books

Goodall, Jane. *Africa in my Blood: An Autobiography in Letters.* New York: Houghton Mifflin, 2000.

———. *Chimpanzees I Love: Saving Their World and Ours.* New York: Scholastic Press, 2001.

———. *In the Shadow of Man.* Boston: Houghton Mifflin, 1971.

———. *My Life with the Chimpanzees.* New York: Byron Preiss Visual Publications, Inc. New York, 1988.

———. *Through a Window: My Thirty Years with the Chimpanzees of Gombe.* Boston: Houghton Mifflin, 1990. (These books chronicle Jane Goodall's four decades of work with the chimpanzees in the northwest region of Tanzania, now the Gombe National Reserve.)

Ridgeway, Rick. *The Shadow of Kilimanjaro: On Foot Across East Africa.* New York: Henry Holt, 1998.

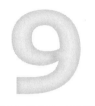

ACHILLES KATAMBA

HENRY LUZZE

JAMES OLOYA

CHRISTOPHER C. WHALEN

UGANDA

The History of Uganda

About 5000 BCE, Bantu-speaking peoples migrated from western Africa to the east-central region now called Uganda. By the fourteenth century AD, three kingdoms dominated the region—Buganda (meaning "state of the Gandas," and the origin of the country's name), Bunyoro, and Ankole. The British colonized Uganda in 1894 and ruled the territory as a British protectorate until 9 October 1962, when Uganda declared its independence. Sir Edward Mutesa, the king of Buganda Kingdom, was elected the first president, and Dr. Milton Apollo Obote became the first prime minister. In 1966, Prime Minister Obote seized control of the government with the help of Colonel Idi Amin.

On 25 January 1971, Colonel Idi Amin deposed President Obote, who sought refuge in the neighboring country of Tanzania. Amin governed the country as a military dictatorship. Shortly after becoming president, he expelled all Indian residents from Uganda. In 1976, he proclaimed himself president for life. In an attempt to annex the Kagara region of Tanzania to Uganda, Amin waged military attacks on the Tanzanian-Uganda border in 1978.[1] As a result of these attacks, a combined force of Tanzanian troops and Ugandan exiles loyal to former president Obote invaded Uganda and ousted Amin in 1979. Amin went into exile in Saudi Arabia, where he died in 2007.

Two interim administrations led the country before President Obote was returned to power in 1980, after a multiparty election that was tainted by alleged massive vote rigging. Obote was ousted in a military coup by his army commander, General Tito Lutwa, in July 1985. On 26 January 1986, the National Resistance Army, led by Yoweri Museveni, seized power, and Museveni declared himself president of the Republic of Uganda. Since then, most areas of Uganda have prospered from a period of relative peace and steady economic growth. However, Uganda's northern region experienced an eighteen-year-long battle against the brutal Lord's Resistance Army, led by Joseph Kony. The insurgence displaced up to 1.5 million people. As of 2008, peace has returned to the region, and Kony and three of his officers have been indicted on charges of crimes against humanity by the International Criminal Court.

Modern Uganda

Uganda is in East Africa, bordered on the west by the Democratic Republic of Congo, on the north by the Sudan, on the east by Kenya, and on the south by Tanzania and Rwanda. Uganda lies across the equator and is divided into three main types of terrain: swampy lowlands, a fertile plateau with wooded hills, and semi-arid regions. Lake Victoria forms part of the southern border. Uganda is a country of 30.8 million people, with a growth rate of 2.7 percent and a birth rate of 47.8 per 1,000 population. The country's infant mortality rate is 65 per 1,000 live births. Life expectancy is 51.6 years for males and 53.8 years for females. The capital city is Kampala, with a population of 1,461,600.

Economy

Although Uganda is one of the poorest countries in Africa, its economy has been among the fastest growing in sub-Saharan Africa. Building on a foundation of two decades of peace and sound development policies, Uganda has achieved impressive economic growth, low inflation, and steady reduction of poverty.[2] The Gross Domestic Product (GDP; see the glossary) per capita is $1,100, with a real growth rate of 6.9 percent and inflation of 6.8 percent. The country's economy relies mainly on subsistence agriculture and to a lesser extent on high-productivity manufacturing. Its main export earners include coffee, fish and fish products, tea, cotton, flowers, and gold.[3]

Language and Literacy

English is the official language and the language of instruction in schools at all levels in Uganda. However, there are many local languages spoken by different ethnic groups. Luganda (one of the Bantu languages) is the most commonly spoken by people from the central part of the country. Other common languages include Nilo-hamitic, Luo, Swahili, and Arabic. The literacy rate among Ugandans fifteen and older is estimated to be 67 percent, and it is higher among males (77 percent) than females (58 percent).

The Ugandan Education System

The current educational system in Uganda was established in the early 1960s and consists of four levels of education: pre-primary level, followed by seven years of primary education, four to six years of post-primary (secondary) level, and a post-secondary level that includes tertiary education at technical schools or universities.

Pre-primary education is run by private agencies or individuals and provides early education to children two to five years old. Enrollment in pre-primary education is low; only about 10 percent of children complete pre-primary school. Parents or guardians are solely responsible for financing education at this level, although the government provides guidelines outlining a standard curriculum for children and teachers through the Education Act of 2008.

Primary education is universal and compulsory for children ages six and older. In 1997, the government introduced a universal primary education system in which the government pays the tuition fees for all students with the aim of creating equitable access to an affordable quality education for all children regardless of sex, socioeconomic background, or special circumstances. Primary education spans seven years. Though universal in coverage, there are variations in educational opportunities between urban and rural areas; urban areas have more permanent schools, access to larger numbers of teachers with advanced education, and higher-quality instructional materials than do schools in rural areas.

Upon successful completion of primary school, children can enroll in secondary school. Secondary education is six years in length, composed of four years of ordinary secondary and two years of advanced secondary schooling. Only about 40 percent of primary school graduates are absorbed into the secondary school cycle, which may indicate that there are fewer school spaces than available students. Students who success-fully complete the four-year ordinary secondary level then have four possible outlets:

Advanced secondary school;
Technical institutes for a two- or three-year advanced craft course;
Primary teacher college for a two-year course; and
Governmental department training colleges.

Graduates of advanced secondary education have several options de-pending on their performance on advanced level examinations. They can enroll in a university with private or government sponsorship or attend teacher training colleges, business colleges, or vocational institutions.

There are six international schools in Uganda, all located in Kam-pala. These are private institutions offering foreign curricula, examina-tions, and certification. They generally offer pre-primary, primary, and secondary school education.

University Education in Uganda
In the last few years, Uganda has seen an increase in the number of universities in the country. Today, there are five government-sponsored universities (Makerere University, Mbarara University of Science and Technology, Kyambogo University, Gulu University, and Busitema Uni-versity) and twenty-one private universities.

Makerere University was established in 1922 and is one of the oldest and most prestigious universities in Africa. Currently, it has twenty-two faculties, institutes, and schools offering degrees, diplomas, and certifi-cates to a student body of about 30,000 undergraduates and 3,000 post-graduates, both Ugandan and international students. It is the country's leading research institution.

Mbarara University of Science and Technology was founded in 1989, with a mission to provide applied science and technology education. The university offers undergraduate and graduate degrees, diplomas, and certificates. Gulu University, located in northern Uganda, was estab-lished in 2003, and offers teacher education, science, medicine, technol-ogy, business management, rural transformation, and conflict studies. Kyambogo University, just outside Kampala, emphasizes science, tech-nology and education. Busitema University, in the country's eastern re-gion, has an emphasis on agricultural sciences and engineering.

The Ugandan Healthcare System

Structure of the Healthcare System

The government of Uganda, through its Ministry of Health, is responsible for delivering healthcare to Ugandans. It does so through the National Health System (NHS). The NHS is comprised of both public and private healthcare delivery systems made up of hospitals and health centers. Hospitals are located at the district, regional, and national levels. Health centers are categorized from level I through level IV, depending on the size of the population served, from the community or village (I), to the parish (II), subcounty (III), and larger (IV). In each of the eighty administrative districts in Uganda, the district health officer is the head of the District Health Service, which is a self-contained segment of the NHS and includes all actors in the recognized spheres of health in the district.

The health subdistrict is the functional subdivision or service zone of the District Health Service. The subdistrict is mandated to bring essential care closer to the people, allow for identification of local priorities, involve communities in the planning and management of health services, and increase responsiveness to local needs.[4]

Function of the National Health System

The overall function of the NHS is to deliver a minimum healthcare package that addresses communicable diseases — particularly malaria, acute respiratory tract infections, HIV/AIDS, tuberculosis (TB), and diarrheal diseases — and provides services to address malnutrition and perinatal and maternal conditions. Together these conditions continue to account for the overwhelming proportion of disease and premature death among Ugandans.

The Ministry of Health has organized a number of disease-specific programs to control and eliminate common diseases such as malaria, TB, and HIV/AIDS.

The Malaria Control Programme

Malaria is considered endemic (see the glossary) in Uganda.[5] The country's Malaria Control Programme guides the implementation of national malaria control policies to reduce the malaria burden in Uganda. The program facilitates enhanced communication among international partners working on malaria control and the public at large. The program's website contains useful information and data regarding malaria control in Uganda.[6]

The National Tuberculosis and Leprosy Control Programme

TB control efforts in Uganda date back to 1965, when the National Tuberculosis Control Programme was established. The current combined National Tuberculosis and Leprosy Control Programme was started in 1990. The program falls under the jurisdiction of the Department of National Disease Control at the Ministry of Health.[7] It has three operational levels — at the central, district, and health facility levels. At the central level, the program is directed by a program manager, who is assisted by six zonal TB and leprosy supervisors representing the program's six implementing zones. The program's central unit sets policies, generates technical reports, publishes operational guidelines, ensures timely drug procurement, and organizes staff training. At the district level, TB and leprosy control activities are directed by a district TB and leprosy supervisor, who is supervised by the district health officer and the zonal supervisor. The health facility level includes health facilities ranging from Health Center II at the parish, to Health Center III at the subcounty, and Health Center IV at the subdistrict levels, district hospitals at the district level, regional referral hospitals at the regional level, and the national referral hospital at the national level.

HIV/AIDS Control in Uganda

The Uganda AIDS Control Programme was established in 1986. Its early goals were to inform people on how HIV is transmitted, help change high-risk behaviors, and promote non-risk sexual behavior.[8] Early in the HIV epidemic, the government of Uganda realized that the epidemic affected all sectors of society and could not be controlled by the Ministry of Health alone. Thus, the government established the Uganda AIDS Commission in 1992, as a multisectoral corporate body housed in the president's office, with a broader mission.[9]

The functions of the Uganda AIDS Commission are broad and multifaceted, and they include all areas of policy and program implementation. Because the commission supervises all activities relating to control of the AIDS epidemic, its purview includes: health care and counseling of AIDS patients; the welfare of bereaved orphans and survivors of AIDS victims; provision of medical supplies and equipment; handling of socioeconomic, cultural, and legal issues related to the AIDS epidemic; and biomedical research into and surveillance of the AIDS epidemic and methods of prevention and control.

Regulation of Health Research

The Ministry of Health and the Ministry of Finance, Planning, and Economic Development are responsible for the regulation of health research in Uganda.[10] Two other statutory bodies are also involved: the Uganda National Council of Science and Technology and the Uganda National Health Research Organization, which is responsible for the administration and guidance of the country's research institutions, such as its Cancer Research Institute and its Virus Research Institute, to name just two.

The council is responsible for overseeing all research that occurs in Uganda after it has undergone scientific and ethical approval in academic, research, and development institutions. It acts as a clearinghouse in which all health research is registered. Together with the National Drug Authority, the council evaluates research involving clinical trials of drugs or vaccines, and evaluates the drugs themselves before permits for trials can be issued.

Leading Health and Environmental Issues in Uganda

HIV Infection and AIDS

Uganda was the first country in sub-Saharan Africa to experience and recognize the HIV epidemic. As early as 1982, local healthcare providers, traditional healers, and villagers recognized that young men and women living in the Rakai region of southwestern Uganda were dying of an unknown disease. This disease produced severe wasting and was referred to as *silimi*, or slim disease, by the local community.[11] Families were disrupted, and orphaned children were being taken care of by their grandparents or were adopted by other family members. Entire villages were gutted as the men and women of childbearing and income-earning age died of the disease. No disease in recent history had led to such devastation.

By 1985, public health officials had made the link between the newly discovered Human Immunodeficiency Virus, type 1 (HIV), and slim dis-

ease.[12] With the development of blood tests and the conduct of prevalence surveys for HIV infection, it was clear by 1988 that the country had
been hit hard and early by the HIV epidemic. Surveys in sentinel populations (that is, populations in which surveys were conducted over time)
indicated an unprecedented prevalence of infection. For instance, pregnant mothers attending antenatal clinics had HIV prevalence levels of
25 percent;[13] patients with sexually transmitted diseases had prevalence
levels of 30 percent; and tuberculosis patients had 67 percent HIV prevalence.[14] It was often stated that every citizen of Uganda knew someone
with AIDS or who had died from AIDS. The HIV epidemic threatened
the very fabric of Ugandan culture and endangered a fragile country just
emerging from twenty years of civil wars.

The Ugandan response to the HIV/AIDS epidemic was nothing short
of remarkable. In 1987, Noerine Kaleeba and colleagues founded The
AIDS Support Organization (TASO). This was a national nongovernmental organization (NGO; see the glossary) that provided both Western medicine and traditional healing to patients with AIDS. Apart from
the provision of health care, TASO also provided a place where people
"unified by common experiences faced when encountering HIV/AIDS
at a time of high stigma, ignorance and discrimination"[15] could go for
solace and counseling. Around the same time a popular singer, Philly
Lutaya, was diagnosed with AIDS. He was one of the first Ugandans to
declare his disease and talk openly about his experiences. He traveled
around the country meeting with community leaders, grass-roots organizations, and students at schools, all in an effort to educate people and
destigmatize AIDS. The end result of TASO's efforts and Lutaya's life,
and indeed the decision of the country's president Yoweri Museveni,
was to be open about HIV/AIDS and address the problem directly.

The government has been actively engaged in its response to the HIV/
AIDS epidemic. As mentioned above, the Ministry of Health created the
Uganda AIDS Commission to develop policies for the prevention and
control of HIV/AIDS in the country. A consortium of government and
academic institutions established the Joint Clinical Research Center in
1992, with a threefold mission: to evaluate the extent of the HIV problem in the military; to conduct research on HIV/AIDS prevention and
treatment; and to provide care for patients with AIDS.

The openness on this issue in the country led to a national campaign
of education, counseling, and HIV testing. Even at a time when there

was no treatment, "know your status" was a clear message. In 1990, the AIDS Information Centre was opened in Kampala to provide the first confidential, voluntary counseling and testing center in the country. At the center, clients could receive pre- and post-test counseling, HIV testing, and education about HIV. The demand for HIV testing was so great that the center expanded its services in the city and set up satellite centers throughout the country.

In the absence of, or with very limited access to, antiretroviral therapy (ART; see the glossary), Uganda naturally focused on HIV prevention interventions. The work by TASO and other groups to mitigate stigma and discrimination, the open dialogue encouraged by the Ministry of Health, and the political support of the president all contributed to social change. Widespread availability of voluntary counseling and testing laid the foundation for successful prevention programs. Throughout much of the 1990s, Uganda developed and implemented scientifically based, pragmatic interventions to prevent transmission of HIV. These included school-based education about HIV, peer-based programs, condom promotion, treatment of sexually transmitted diseases, and treatment of pregnant mothers with HIV. These interventions delayed sexual debut, reduced the number of sexual partners, increased the use of condoms, and lowered the incidence of sexually transmitted diseases in the country. The net effect of this vigorous, open, and multi-faceted approach was to reduce HIV prevalence from 21 percent in 1991 to 6.5 percent in 2004-5, as documented by a national HIV seroprevalence survey. The HIV prevalence rate in Uganda is now approximately 5.4 percent, one of the lowest rates in Africa. Uganda's multisectoral response and, in a sense, its "success story" have provided a hopeful and important example for its East African neighbors and, indeed, all of sub-Saharan Africa.

Although Ugandan health officials were pleased with HIV prevention progress, they were keenly aware of the developments in effective treatment and aggressively sought ways to introduce ART into Uganda. As early as 1995, the Joint Clinical Research Center was evaluating the role of azidothymidine (AZT) in small clinical trials. However, prior to 1996, when the protease inhibitors were first released, the overall effectiveness of mono- or duo-therapy for HIV was minimal, and there was little demand for these expensive medications in Africa. Following the historic international AIDS meeting in Durban, South Africa in

1998, the demands for access to the new, potent, and expensive antiretroviral medications in Africa grew louder. In 2003, several large international donors provided the financial support to rapidly expand and scale up treatment and prevention efforts in Africa. The largest program to date is the President's Emergency Plan for AIDS Relief (PEPFAR; see the glossary). PEPFAR provides funding to support the treatment of HIV in many countries of Africa, including Uganda. Since 2004, Uganda has received $929 million to support a comprehensive HIV/AIDS care, treatment, and prevention program,[16] which has increased treatment, testing, counseling, and exposure to prevention. To date, over 150,000 people with AIDS are receiving lifelong ART. As of 2008, some 400,000 HIV-positive individuals have received care for HIV; over four million counseling and testing encounters have occurred; 100,000 pregnant women have received prophylactic therapy for the prevention of mother-to-child-transmission; and over six million Ugandans have heard or participated in HIV prevention programs.

As part of its broad-based response to the HIV/AIDS epidemic, Uganda has pursued basic, clinical, and epidemiologic research on HIV/AIDS. As a strategy, Ugandan scientists and health officials formed international collaborations with leading U.S. and European institutions, engaging in cutting-edge research on HIV prevention, mother-to-child transmission, and HIV-TB interactions. This research not only provided key information needed to formulate health policy in the country, but also led to technology transfer and capacity building. The country now has sophisticated laboratories with state-of-the-art technologies in which national and international researchers come together to study HIV and its complications at the Joint Clinical Research Center, in Kampala, and the Uganda Virus Research Institute, in Entebbe. We describe some of these international collaborations later in this chapter.

Today, the full spectrum of HIV preventive and medical care is available to Uganda's citizens. Despite the progress in improved access to ART, the country still remains vulnerable to HIV/AIDS. Challenges posed by a mature AIDS epidemic include morbidity and mortality related to AIDS and its associated opportunistic infections, the commonest of which is TB. Antiretroviral drug resistance is an anticipated consequence of wider access to these medications. A range of strategies are being undertaken to address these challenges: strengthening prevention strategies; implementing new, effective interventions in ART delivery and HIV care; and addressing gaps in clinical, operational, health services, and implementation research. There is a need to scale up interventions and increase access to ART to reach marginal populations in rural areas of the country. There is now an urgent need to implement evidence-based practices related to chronic HIV care and address barriers in the Ugandan healthcare context, which is still characterized by limited resources and a weak health system.

Tuberculosis

TB is an ancient disease that continues to threaten both individual and public health throughout the world. Although it is both a treatable and preventable condition, current public health strategies have failed to control the disease in many parts of the world, especially in the developing countries of sub-Saharan Africa. In these countries, the problem of TB is compounded by the HIV epidemic, the emergence of multidrug-resistant TB (MDR TB; see the glossary), and the limited effectiveness of TB control programs. In Uganda, like the rest of sub-Saharan Africa, tuberculosis remains a scourge today.

Historically, TB was present in the region of Uganda around Lake Victoria by the end of the nineteenth century. In medical records maintained by Sir Albert Cook, a British physician and explorer, clinical cases of tuberculosis were described in detail.[17] In 1965, shortly after Uganda gained its independence from Britain, the country launched a national tuberculosis program to control TB, consistent with recommendations from the World Health Organization (WHO; see the glossary). However, during the years of civil war, TB control was abandoned and health records were not maintained. In 1988, tuberculosis and leprosy control efforts were merged to form the current National Tuberculosis and Leprosy Control Programme (described earlier in this chapter), and by the early 1990s, the program had established surveillance capacity and begun keeping national statistics.

Even before the HIV epidemic, TB was endemic in Uganda. The greatest burden of disease was in cities where poverty contributed to overcrowding and TB transmission. Healthcare providers who saw patients during the turbulent decades of the 1970s and 1980s described TB as a common but not overwhelming condition, until the HIV epidemic seized the country. With the HIV epidemic, rates of TB rose dramatically, and the tuberculosis wards of hospitals around the country began to fill up. Indeed, the sharp rise in TB rates was one of the initial indicators of the HIV epidemic in Uganda, as many of the patients with slim disease had tuberculosis. Soon, more than two-thirds of TB patients presenting to the National Tuberculosis and Leprosy Control Programme were infected with HIV.[18] Mortality from HIV-associated TB approached 20 percent in the first year after infection with TB, even with effective antituberculosis therapy.[19] TB also seemed to accelerate the clinical course of HIV infection, especially in patients with preserved immunity. The country found itself gripped by another epidemic that was fueled by the HIV epidemic.

In 1993, WHO declared tuberculosis a global emergency, and rolled out DOTS (see the glossary). Over the following years, Uganda systematically developed the capacity to deliver DOTS in accordance with WHO guidelines. The country's current TB control strategy utilizes community health workers located in the villages to observe patient therapy and ensure adherence. Although the country has made great strides in its capacity to control TB, the disease incidence continues to climb. The current incidence rate of new cases of TB in Uganda is estimated to be 330 per 100,000 population.[20] The National Tuberculosis and Leprosy Control Programme continues to be challenged by the high rates of disease, shortages of trained staff, intermittent drug shortages, and limited resources for TB control.

Malaria

Malaria is highly endemic in most parts of Uganda, with climatic conditions that are suitable for transmission of malaria throughout the year. Consequently, 63 percent of the population is exposed to high and 25 percent to moderate malaria transmission levels, while 12 percent live in areas with low or unstable transmission. Areas with low or unstable transmission are regions of the county at altitudes above 1,800 meters (or more than 1 mile), the southwest, the slopes of Mount Elgon, and the Rwenzori mountains, but these areas are prone to periodic malaria outbreaks. Malaria is the leading cause of death among children in Uganda. It is estimated that 70,000–100,000 deaths occur each year among children under five, and between ten and twelve million clinical cases are treated in the public health system alone.[21]

All four human plasmodia species occur in Uganda (see malaria in the glossary), but *Plasmodium falciparum* is by far the most common, contributing 90 percent to 98 percent of the parasite population. The second most common species is *P. malariae*, with 1 percent to 3 percent as mono-infection, but it is more commonly found as a mixed infection with *P. falciparum*, contributing up to 16 percent of childhood infections in highly endemic areas. The second most common species is *P. malariae*, responsible for up to 3 percent of the cases of malaria involving a single parasite and, in combination with *P. falciparum*, for up to 16 percent of childhood infections in highly endemic areas. Both *P. vivax* and *P. ovale* are rare, together accounting for no more than 1.5 percent of malaria cases. Malaria is a vector-borne disease; certain genera of Anopheles mosquitos are the vector. The most common vectors are *Anopheles gambiae* and *A. funestus*, with *A. gambiae* being the dominant species in most places and *A. funestus* found more frequently at higher altitudes. During the short dry seasons, permanent bodies of water are often the most common breeding sites for mosquitoes.

In 1998, the global campaign called Roll Back Malaria was begun. As part of this campaign, Uganda's Malaria Control Programme implemented a strategic plan to control malaria in Uganda by 2009–10, built around the following components: prompt and effective treatment for malaria; vector control, including insecticide-treated bed nets and indoor residual spraying; intermittent preventive treatment during pregnancy; and epidemic preparedness. The program focuses on the accurate and timely clinical and parasitological diagnosis of malaria, followed by treatment with effective antimalarial medications. The program does not focus on treatment alone but offers a package of services that include both treatment and prevention, so that all aspects of malaria control are simultaneously and comprehensively addressed. Efforts are currently under way to expand the coverage with preventive measures to all sectors of Ugandan society. Special efforts are made to reach vulnerable populations such as young children, pregnant women, the economically disadvantaged, people living with HIV/AIDS, and difficult to reach populations such as nomads.

In the years since the Roll Back Malaria campaign began, the incidence of malaria has increased, along with the attendant complications such as malaria-associated deaths, malaria outpatient visits, and malaria hospitalizations. The current incidence of malaria is approximately 488 reported cases per 1,000 population. Whether this represents worsening of the malaria epidemic or improvements in diagnosis and reporting time will tell, as the Uganda Malaria Control Programme closely monitors malaria in the country.

Zoonotic Infections

Zoonoses are defined as those diseases and infections naturally transmitted between people and vertebrate animals. Most zoonotic agents that are endemic in Uganda today are those that have lingered on or have been neglected over time, are endemic in the rural livestock and communities, and are perpetuated by poverty.[22] Classical zoonoses such as bovine tuberculosis, brucellosis, anthrax, and rabies have been reported in pastoral cattle in rural areas in Uganda, and minimal attempts have been made to control them. Most rural communities in Uganda keep livestock for food security, while pastoral communities do so as the source of their livelihood. Agricultural and pastoral occupations are the mainstays of Ugandan economic activity and employment, which puts many people at higher risk of infection with zoonotic agents.

Infections with bovine tuberculosis, brucellosis, Q-fever, leishmaniasis, anthrax, and zoonotic trypanosomiasis in rural areas tend to be occupational, afflicting people of specific ages and genders due to their roles in livestock management. Food-borne infections are believed to be common, but little is known or reported about them. Uganda does not have strong laws or resources to investigate or research zoonotic food-borne infections. Zoonotic infections are not restricted to people in endemic pastoral areas, however. A study of human brucellosis prevalence in Kampala reported that most brucellosis cases in the city resulted from consumption of raw milk transported from periurban or rural areas.[23]

Annual abattoir reports confirm the existence of visible lesions in slaughtered cattle characteristic of some zoonotic agents isolated in pastoral or rural communities. Bovine tuberculosis and brucellosis have been reported in western and midwestern cattle-rearing districts of Uganda. Cases of human infections with the same agents in the same areas as livestock have been reported. Previous studies in pastoral areas in western Uganda reported 74.1 percent of the herds in the region had at least one animal positive to bovine tuberculosis and 55.6 percent to brucellosis,[24] while 13 percent of the goat herds in the eastern region were positive for brucellosis.[25] Dogs, a common grazing and guarding companion in pastoral communities, could play a significant role as a reservoir of infection for the population. They are fed dead, condemned tissues, thus making them potential reservoirs for zoonoses. Because dogs are rarely immunized or dewormed, they are more likely to get rabies or carry echnococcus worms.

The impact of zoonotic infections on rural livestock and the health of the human community that is in close contact with and largely dependent on them as a source of food and livelihood is not entirely known. A study of lymph node biopsies of patients with cervical lymphadenitis reporting for TB treatment in the pastoral areas of northeastern Uganda showed 6.9 percent of isolates being *Mycobacterium bovis*.[26] A study on the etiology of low back pain in Mulago hospital reported 5.9 percent of cases were due to brucella,[27] suggesting that the problem could be bigger than reported. Zoonoses commonly diagnosed in urban health centers in Uganda have been traced to patients from rural areas who seek treatment in the city or to consumption of animal products originating from rural areas.

Most zoonoses have specific endemic areas. For example, bovine tuberculosis, brucellosis, dog rabies, and parasitic conditions such as cysticercosis, taeniasis, and echinoccosis are endemic in pastoral communities in Karamoja (in the northeastern region), the central region, and western Uganda. Cysticercosis, echinococcosis, and leishmaniasis are endemic in both livestock and humans in the Karamoja region. Zoonotic trypanosomoses is endemic in cattle and people in the eastern region (Busoga and Teso regions), while seasonal rabies outbreaks are common in dogs in most districts of Uganda. Other zoonotic infections like salmonellosis, *E. coli*, shigellosis, trematodiasis, Q-fever, and toxoplasmosis are less frequently reported or not reported at all. Highly pathogenic but rarer zoonoses such as hepatitis E, plague, and Ebola and Marburg hemorrhagic fevers attract attention and draw swift response from the government and donor funding agencies. Often the response to less dramatically pathogenic zooneses is less vigorous.

The usually low mortality rates from zoonotic diseases mean that they may not receive heightened attention. In cases of brucellosis, for instance, symptoms such as fever, headache, and malaise are similar to many other ailments such as malaria and tend to be mistaken or overlooked. Many residents in rural communities are also too poor to seek services from health centers. A logistical problem in the control of zoonoses is that these are diseases that require the involvement of both medical and veterinary expertise for their control. Zoonoses control in Uganda falls in the gap between veterinary and medical responsibilities, and human medical needs often end up getting overlooked. Measures to safeguard human health and to control disease in livestock to prevent transmission of zoonotic diseases are too often undertaken in isolation from one another. The frequently understaffed and underfunded veterinary and medical departments within the Ministry of Health each hope that the other will deal with the problem, and each department carries out its operations separately, limiting effective and coordinated planning.

Global Health Agencies and Initiatives in Uganda

The breadth of projects and initiatives currently being undertaken in Uganda is vast. Governmental agencies and NGOs, each with its own special interest and emphasis, carry out a large range of activities. The agencies and programs listed below should not be considered comprehensive, but a sample of some of the groups currently engaged in global health work in Uganda.

International and National Institutions

WHO is the coordinating authority for health within the United Nations system. It provides leadership on global health—setting norms and standards of health care, providing technical support to a country, and monitoring and assessing health trends. The WHO mission in Uganda assists the country in achieving the Millennium Development Goals (MDGS; see the glossary). It is coordinated through the Regional Office for Africa and implements central WHO policy and coordinates programs in the country.

The U.S. Centers for Disease Control and Prevention (CDC) has a Center on Global Health that extends its knowledge and activities to promote health around the world. The CDC offices in Uganda are located at the Uganda Virus Research Institute, in Entebbe. One of the CDC's main programs is the Global AIDS Program. Launched in 2000, its activities in Uganda are centered on prevention of HIV transmission, care and treatment of those already infected, and laboratory services and capacity building.

The Infectious Disease Institute is an NGO run by Makerere University and launched with support from Pfizer, Inc. The institute envisions an Africa free from the burdens of infectious diseases. It is dedicated to building the capacity of health systems in Africa for the delivery of sustainable, high-quality healthcare and prevention of HIV/AIDS and related infections, training future clinicians and scientists, and enabling cutting-edge research and clinical services. It has formed partnerships with the Ugandan Ministries of Health and Education, the Uganda AIDS Commission, the Kampala City Council, and foreign institutions such as the Academic Alliance.

The Medical Research Council research unit on AIDS in Uganda is based at the Uganda Virus Research Institute, on the shores of Lake Victoria in Entebbe, and has three field stations in Masaka and Jinja districts. The unit was established following a 1988 request from the Ugandan government to the British government for assistance in research and control of HIV infection and AIDS. Reflecting the wide-ranging nature of the problems caused by HIV, it is multidisciplinary in approach. Its primary focus is to investigate HIV infection-related issues of public health relevance to Uganda and other parts of sub-Saharan Africa. With capacities ranging from virology and immunology to social science, clinical studies, and intervention trials, its research activities encompass five main areas: (1) observational studies of the epidemiology, clinical characteristics, and determinants of the HIV epidemic in the presence of care; (2) research to identify and evaluate interventions to reduce HIV transmission; (3) research to develop and evaluate interventions to reduce disease progression; (4) studies of the behavioral aspects of prevention and care and the social consequences of the epidemic; and (5) basic science research on the development of vaccines and issues of viral resistance to antiretroviral drugs.

Foreign Academic Institutions

Since the end of civil strife in Uganda in 1986, academic institutions from the United States and Europe have played important roles in rebuilding government universities, technical schools, and training programs. The following universities have a strong presence in the country.

The Uganda–Case Western Research Collaboration was formed in 1987, after Frederick C. Robbins — a professor, dean emeritus, and Nobel laureate — and other faculty members from Case Western Reserve University visited Uganda to assess the HIV/AIDS epidemic and assist the Ugandan Ministry of Health in developing a research agenda.

The formal collaboration between Case Western, Makerere University, and the Ugandan Ministry of Health began in August 1988, with support from an International Collaboration for AIDS Research grant and an AIDS International Training and Research training grant from the Fogarty International Center of the U.S. National Institutes of Health. The following years saw rapid growth in research activities in Uganda. A central tenet of this rapidly growing, vibrant collaboration has been the integration of training and research in order to build scientific and technical capacity in the country. Now in its twenty-first year, the collaboration has enabled over fifty Ugandan scientists, physicians, and public health officials to get advanced degrees in epidemiology, microbiology, molecular biology, virology, immunology, or anthropology. Graduates of this program have returned to Uganda to become leaders in government, clinical care, and education.

The research agenda of the Uganda–Case Western Research Collaboration emerged historically through a matching of the exigent needs in Uganda and the expertise at Case. The research includes: the substantive and long-term study of HIV and its interactions with TB; strategies for HIV prevention, treatment, and care; and basic virology. To accomplish the research goals, investigators have built research capacity by developing modern laboratories in immunology, virology, molecular biology, and clinical chemistry, located at the Joint Clinical Research Center and Makerere University. These projects, and the infrastructure they have spawned, provide a foundation for patient-oriented research and training for the future.

The University of California, San Francisco started to work in Uganda in the early 1990s, initially supporting American clinicians as they lived, worked, and taught at Mulago Hospital. Research efforts spanned such areas as sexually transmitted diseases, cryptococcal meningitis, and malaria in Uganda, focusing on the evaluation of novel therapies in children, and later on the effect of coinfection with HIV. Today, this collaboration between the U.S. university and the Ugandan hospital encompasses a broad array of studies, from evaluating novel approaches to HIV testing in TB patients, to optimal delivery of ART in rural regions of the country.

The collaboration between Uganda and Johns Hopkins University began in 1987. With a small start-up grant from the U.S. Agency for International Development (USAID; see the glossary), David Serwadda, Nelson Sewankambo, and Maria Wawer began to study the HIV epidemic in the Rakai district, located in the southwestern part of the country. The Rakai Health Sciences Program was launched and rapidly grew into one of the most successful examples of international collaboration. This group leads the world in its population-based research on HIV transmission. Some of the important findings to come out of their collaborative research include: that viral load is a key determinant in the likelihood of HIV transmission; that reducing sexually transmitted diseases does not lessen HIV incidence in communities with a mature, generalized epidemic; and that circumcised men are less likely to be infected with HIV. In 1996, Brooks Jackson joined the faculty with a successful research program on the prevention of mother-to-child HIV transmission at Mulago Hospital. He has since expanded his research program to include testing new HIV vaccines and has developed an accredited clinical laboratory in the Makerere Medical School. Today, the extensive collaboration between Makerere University and Johns Hopkins University targets many new areas in clinical care, education, and research; the questions the collaboration addresses continue to have implications for disease control and health policy worldwide.

Conclusion

In Uganda, as in many African countries, there is a clash between the traditions of Africa and the growing presence of Western culture. This may best be appreciated in the contrast between life in a city like Kampala and life in a neighboring village. Kampala is a large, dynamic, and busy city with its business district, industrial areas, fancy shopping centers, grocery stores, electronics shops, wonderful restaurants, and sites for evening entertainment. Kampala is also home to Makerere University's main campus and its newly reorganized College of Health Sciences. There are hospitals, clinics, and pharmacies that can provide high-quality medical care for those who can afford it. The streets are filled with cars, buses, *boda-bodas* (motorbikes), *matatus* (minibuses), bicycles, and pedestrians. And endless traffic jams. On the hills surrounding the city, there are churches of many denominations and mosques. People are going about the business of their day, wearing professional attire, carrying briefcases, talking and texting on their cell phones. If it weren't for the GPS coordinates on your cell phone, you might think you were in a bustling European city.

If you were to catch a ride out of town on a *boda-boda*, within minutes you would arrive in the surrounding residential neighborhoods of single-family homes, apartment complexes, and an occasional shanty town. Here you won't find large stores and businesses, but rather small, family-owned shops and stores. There are butcher shops with carcasses hanging on display, fish vendors with their catch of the day, chickens caged and stacked. In front of and between these shops, individuals will sell the fruits and vegetables that they do not need that day. Your eye will be caught by the enormous piles of plantains that are balanced on the back of bicycles. Neat pyramids of tomatoes, bushels of large green avocados, boxes of freshly cut pineapple are displayed and tended to by an eager salesperson. There are also shops that sell grains and rice, usually stored in fifty-pound bags and carefully weighed out on a hanging scale at the time of purchase. Interspersed are small pharmacies, general stores, stationery stores, beauty salons, gas stations, and bars.

As you move away from the main road, usually on a bumpy dirt road, and travel for several kilometers, you will leave behind the sights and sounds of the city and move into the real Africa, the rural part of the continent where most Africans live, and where African tradition still affects all aspects of life. Instead of tightly packed buildings made out of clay bricks, stucco siding, and corrugated metal roofs, you will see small homes made of wood, daub, mud, and wattle, with thatched roofs. Often these modest homes are grouped in a compound of three or four related families. Together with neighboring compounds and houses, this is an African village. The pace of life in the village appears slower and more relaxed, though the villagers are no less busy than their counterparts in the city. Their daily life is about subsistence, growing enough crops and raising enough poultry or cattle or pigs to feed their family. If they are fortunate, they will sell the extra at the nearby trading center. Unlike in the city, children and parents are together. Mothers tend to their chores with infants on their backs. Older children play beside their mothers, and still older ones help with the chores. There are large jerrycans (large, usually yellow plastic containers) that hold the day's supply of fresh water. The air is filled with the smell of charcoal from the small fires that are kept burning throughout the day.

Despite the modernization of Uganda, its culture is dominated by tribal traditions. There are fifty-three different tribes in Uganda; the largest one, which dominates the culture in and around Kampala, is the Baganda tribe. Before the civil wars, when the Ugandan government abolished all kingdoms, the Baganda were organized as a kingdom, headed by the *kabaka*, or king. In 1993, the kingdom was restored, and the *kabaka* returned to Uganda for the first time since 1967. The center of the kingdom is the Kasubi tombs, where past kings are buried and where elders maintain their folklore in the form of myths, legends, and proverbs.

Tribal beliefs shape family and social relationships, including choice of a spouse in marriage, religious choices, business partnerships, and even local enemies and villains. In this tribe and others, there is a profound respect for elders. This respect underlies the structure of Ugandan society and affects all interactions, whether in personal or professional spheres. Major decisions and actions of a family or clan must have the blessings of the elder, chief, or head of that family. Similarly, in a professional transaction, the head of a business or project must be informed of all activities and decisions, including the decision to allow a visitor to see or tour the project, or to allow a volunteer to work in the business or project. To show respect for the culture, a global health student or worker must first introduce himself or herself to the "elder" of a project or activity. In the introduction, the student should present qualifications, discuss the goals and aims of his or her work on the project, and formally request permission to be part of the project. It is often a good idea for a student to be introduced by a person known by the elder or head, as this adds a vote of confidence in the student's involvement.

Uganda is a former British protectorate that gained its independence in 1962, but soon fell into civil war that decimated the nascent political, economic, and health infrastructure in the country. Over the past twenty years, however, Uganda has experienced political stability and strong leadership that has led the country out of the turmoil of civil strife to become one of the most dynamic and vibrant countries in Africa. What is most remarkable is that this growth and development has occurred in the face of the devastating epidemics of HIV/AIDS, TB, and malaria. Although the country's economy has grown and modernized, it is not yet able to sustain all government functions. As a result, Uganda has entered into formative partnerships with NGOS, foreign academic institutions, and other foreign partners to sustain and build in the areas of healthcare, education, and agriculture, to name only a few. The future for Uganda is bright, though to stay the current course, it will take lead-

ership that is committed to a fair political process and a strong commitment to progress through partnership.

APPENDIX

COUNTRY DATA : UGANDA

Millennium Development Goal indicators are italicized.

TABLE 9.1 : **POPULATION AND HUMAN DEVELOPMENT**

POPULATION	
Total	30.8 million
Population growth rate	2.7%
Net migration rate/1,000 population	−8.83
Urban	13%
Rural	87%
AGE STRUCTURE	
0–14 years	50.0%
15–64 years	47.9%
65+ years	2.1%
Median age (years)	15
MAJOR ETHNIC GROUPS	
Baganda	17%
Bankayole	9.5%
Basoga	8.4%
Bakiga	7.0%
Other	58.3%
RELIGIONS	
Roman Catholic	41.9%
Protestant	42.0%
Muslim	12.1%
Other	3.1%
None	0.9%
HUMAN DEVELOPMENT	
Human Development Index	0.505
Human Development rank[a]	154th
Freedom House Index	Partly free
Political Rights score[b]	5
Civil Liberties score[b]	4
Human Poverty Index	34.7%
Human Poverty rank[c]	154th

Notes: [a]out of 179 countries; [b]1 = most free, 7 = least free; [c]out of 177 countries

TABLE 9.2 : **GOVERNMENT AND ECONOMY**

GOVERNMENT	
Independence	9 Oct.1962 from Britain
Type of government	Republic
Voting rights	Age 18, universal
CAPITAL	Kampala
CURRENCY	Ugandan Shilling (UGX)
ECONOMY	
Gross domestic product (GDP) (in PPP US $)	$35.88 billion
Annual GDP growth	6.9%
GDP per capita (in US $)	$1,100
Annual GDP growth	6.9%
Gini Index	45.7
Population living below PPP $1/day	51.5%
External debt service as % of GDP	2.0
Public debt as % of GDP	17.4
Official development assistance (ODA) per capita (in US $)	$41.6
Foreign direct investment as % of GDP	2.9
LABOR FORCE	
In agriculture	82%
In industry	5%
In services	13%
Unemployment rate	3.2%

TABLE 9.3 : **GEOGRAPHY AND ENVIRONMENT**

LAND COMPOSITION

Land area	241,038 sq. km. (93,065 sq. mi.)
Size comparison	Slightly smaller than Oregon
Terrain	Mostly plateau with rim of mountains; fertile, with many lakes and rivers, landlocked
Ecological hazards	NA

LAND USE AND RESOURCES

Permanent crop land	8.9%
Arable land	21.6%
Agricultural products	Coffee, tea, cotton, tobacco, cassava, potatoes, corn, millet, cut flowers, meat, poultry, milk
Natural resources	Copper, cobalt, hydropower, limestone, salt
ENVIRONMENTAL ISSUES	Draining wetlands for agricultural use, deforestation, overgrazing, soil erosion, poaching, hyacinth infestation in Lake Victoria

INFRASTRUCTURE

Population with access to improved water source	*60%*
Population using improved sanitation	*33%*
Roadways unpaved	81%

TABLE 9.4 : **HEALTH**

LIFE, BIRTH, DEATH

    Life expectancy at birth (male/female)   51.6/53.8

    Birth rate/1,000 population   47.84

    Death rate/1,000 population   12.09

    Infant mortality rate/1,000 live births   64.82

PERSONNEL AND INFRASTRUCTURE

    Physicians/100,000 population   8

    Hospital beds/10,000 population   11

HEALTH ECONOMICS

    Total expenditure on health per capita (PPP US $) $135

    Public expenditure on health as % of GDP   2.5

DISEASES

    Most common vector-borne diseases   Malaria, plague, African trypanosomiasis

    Most common food- and water-borne diseases   Bacterial diarrhea, hepatitis A, typhoid fever, schistomosomiasis

    TB incidence/100,000 population   *330*

    TB prevalence/100,000 population   *426*

    New TB cases HIV-positive   39%

    New TB cases multidrug-resistant (MDR)   0.5

    1-year-olds fully immunized against TB   90%

    Estimated malaria cases annually   10.6 million

    Malaria death rate/100,000 population   0.99

    HIV prevalence rate in adults   *5.4%*

    AIDS deaths in adults annually   *77,000*

    People living with HIV   940,000

    AIDS orphans   NA

MATERNAL HEALTH

    Fertility rate (children born per woman)   6.77

    Contraceptive prevalence rate (married women 15–49)   *23.7%*

    Maternal mortality rate/100,000 births   *550*

    Lifetime risk of maternal death, 1 in: *25*

    Births attended by skilled birth attendant   *42.1%*

CHILD HEALTH

    Mortality rate of children < 5/1,000 live births   *130*

    1-year olds immunized against measles   *68%*

    Children < 5 using insecticide-treated bed nets   *9.7%*

Children < 5 with fever treated with antimalarial drugs	*61.8%*
Newborns protected against tetanus	86%
HUNGER AND MALNUTRITION	
Children < 5 underweight for age	*20.4%*
Children < 5 under height for age	*45%*
Population undernourished	*19%*

TABLE 9.5 : **LANGUAGE, EDUCATION, AND LITERACY**

LANGUAGES	
English	Official national language
Ganda/Luganda	
Swahili	
Arabic	
Others, including Nil-hamitic, Luo, Swahili	
LITERACY	
Adult literacy rate (population age 15+ who can read and write)	*66.8%*
EXPENDITURE	
Public expenditure on education as % of GDP	5.2
EDUCATION	
Primary mandatory	Yes
Secondary mandatory	No
Net enrollment in primary education[d]	*94.7%*
School life expectancy, in years (male/female)[e]	11/10

[d]Net enrollment rate in primary education is measured as the number of children of official primary school age who are enrolled in primary education as a percentage of children in the official primary school age population.

[e]School life expectancy is the total number of years of school (from primary through tertiary education) that a child can expect to receive.

Principal Sources for Data in Appendix Tables 9.1–9.5

Central Intelligence Agency, *The World Factbook* (https://www.cia.gov/library/publications/the-world-factbook/).

UNDP Human Development Report, 2007/2008, available at: www.hdrstats.undp.org.

UN Millennium Development Goals Indicators Database, available at: www.mdgs.un.org.

UNICEF. The State of the World's Children 2009. Available at: http://www.data.un.org.

WHO. Global Tuberculosis Control. Country Profile: Uganda. WHO Report 2009.

1. The Tanzanian perspective on these events is discussed in the chapter on Tanzania.

2. International Monetary Fund, "IMF Executive Board Concludes 2008 Article IV Consultation with Uganda," Public Information Notice No. 09/23, Washington, D.C.: International Monetary Fund, 23 February 2009 (http://www .imf.org/external/np/sec/pn/2009/pn0923.htm).

3. Central Intelligence Agency, The World Factbook. Uganda (https://www .cia.gov/library/publications/the-world-factbook/geos/ug.html).

4. The Republic of Uganda, Ministry of Health. "Health Sector Strategic Plan II, 2005/06 — 2009/10." July 2005. (http://www.hrhresourcecenter.org/ node/2808).

5. Roll Back Malaria, World Health Organization, and UNICEF, "World Malaria Report 2005," Geneva: World Health Organization, May 2005 (whqlibdoc .who.int/publications/2005/9241593199_eng.pdf).

6. Ministry of Health, The Republic of Uganda, Malaria Control Programme (http://www.health.go.ug/mcp/index2.html).

7. A. Nkolo and S. Kalyesubula-Kibuuka, "Tour of the Districts in the Eastern Zone of Uganda. Activity Report, 12 to 23 December 2005." Kumi, Uganda: The National TB and Leprosy Program, 3 January 2006 (www.kumihospital.org/ reports/ZTLS%20East%2005.doc).

8. F. Elangot, "Uganda: An AIDS Control Programme," AIDS Action, 1, no. 6 (1987): 6 (http://www.ncbi.nlm.nih.gov/pubmed/12341935).

9. Uganda AIDS Commission Act 1992, chap. 208, 13 March 1992.

10. Council for Health Research for Development, COHRED, "Alignment and Harmonization in Health Research: AHA Study, Uganda. Country Report, 2008," Geneva: Council for Health Research for Development, 2008 (www .cohred.org/HRWeb/CMS/pdf/Uganda_web.pdf).

11. D. Serwadda et al., "Slim Disease: A New Disease in Uganda and Its Association with HTLV III Infection," Lancet 19, no.2; (1985): 849–52.

12. Ibid.

13. W. L. Kirungi et al., "Trends in Antenatal HIV Prevalence in Urban Uganda Associated with Uptake of Preventive Sexual Behaviour," Sexually Transmitted Infections 82, supplement 1 (2006): 136–41.

14. P. P. Eriki et al., "The Influence of Human Immunodeficiency Virus Infection on Tuberculosis in Kampala, Uganda," American Review of Respiratory Disease 143 (1991): 185–87.

15. The AIDS Support Organization (TASO), "What Is TASO?" (http://www .tasouganda.org/index.php?option=com_content&view=article&id=44:brief -background&catid=34:taso-background).

16. U.S. President's Emergency Plan for AIDS Relief, FY2008 Country Profile: Uganda (http://www.pepfar.gov/press/countries/profiles/116321.html).

17. T. M. Daniel, "The Early History of Tuberculosis in Central East Africa: Insights from the Clinical Records of the First Twenty Years of Mengo Hospital and Review of Relevant Literature," *International Journal of Tuberculosis and Lung Disease* 2 (1998): 784-90.

18. Ibid.

19. C. C. Whalen et al., "Predictors of Survival in Human Immunodeficiency Virus-infected Patients with Pulmonary Tuberculosis," *American Journal of Respiratory and Critical Care Medicine* 153 (1996): 1977-81.

20. WHO, Global Tuberculosis Control, Country Profile: Uganda, WHO Report 2009 (www.who.int/GlobalAtlas/predefinedReports/TB/PDF_files/uga .pdf).

21. Malaria Control Programme, Ministry of Health, "Uganda Malaria Control Strategy 2005/6-2009/10," p. 6 (www.eac.int/health/index.php?option=com _docman&task=doc). Then go to EAC Public Health Malaria Resource Center to obtain downloadable version of Uganda Malaria Control Strategic Plan.

22. World Health Organization/United Kingdom Department for International Development-Animal Health Programme, (WHO/DFID-HP), "The Control of Neglected Zoonotic Diseases: A Route to Poverty Alleviation. Report of a joint WHO/DFID-AHD Meeting, Geneva, 20 and 21 September 2005," (Geneva: WHO, 2006; www.who.int/zoonoses/Report_Sept06.pdf).

23. K. Makita et al., "Human Brucellosis in Urban and Peri-urban Areas of Kampala, Uganda," *Annals of the New York Academy of Sciences* 1149 (2008): 309-11.

24. F. Bernard et al., "Tuberculosis and Brucellosis Prevalence Survey on Dairy Cattle in Mbarara Milk Basin (Uganda)," *Preventive Veterinary Medicine* 67 (2005): 267-81.

25. E. K. Kabagambe et al., "Risk Factors for Brucella Seropositivity in Goat Herds in Eastern and Western Uganda," *Preventive Veterinary Medicine* 52 (2001): 91-108.

26. J. Oloya et al., "Mycobacteria Causing Human Cervical Lymphadenitis in Pastoral Communities in the Karamoja Region of Uganda," *Epidemiology and Infection* 136 (2008): 636-43.

27. M. Galukande, S. Muwazi, and D. B. Mugisa, "Aetiology of Low Back Pain in Mulago Hospital, Uganda," *African Health Sciences* 5 (2005): 164-67.

LISA V. ADAMS

LAUREL A. SPIELBERG

10

CONCLUDING THOUGHTS

We conclude this book with a few brief thoughts to enhance the experience that your African travels can afford you.

Maximizing Your African Experience

We have learned a number of techniques from our own students who travel to Africa. Integrating these techniques into your plans can lead to a more meaningful travel and work experience, aid a smoother transition when you return from Africa, and build on the work you do while there. These techniques include: setting goals for your experience; enhancing your communication skills; working with an identified advisor or mentor; sharing your experiences both while in Africa and after your return home; extending your learning; and building on your experiences for future endeavors or career choices.

Set Goals for Your African Experience

Preparing a set of goals for your African experience is a key step in planning a meaningful venture. Your goals may be simple and singular, or numerous and varied. You might aim to learn basic communication skills in the language of your destination country, have a hands-on experience working with local health providers or other experts in your area of interest, learn how colleagues with your career goals are trained in the country, or carry out a specific project that entails gathering or analyzing data or implementing a new program. In working towards your goals it's important to remain flexible, open to unplanned opportunities, and resilient in the face of disappointment or change.

In the spirit of promoting partnership as the foundation of any endeavor you undertake in Africa, we offer the following additional bit of cautionary advice about the goals of your undertaking. Understandably, many students and volunteer workers depart for Africa with a strong motivation to help others in need, to make a significant contribution to a greater public health goal, or to have a meaningful impact in the country where they will be working. Our experiences mentoring students on global health internships have given us a highly realistic perspective: you should realize that in all likelihood *you* are the one who will gain the most from this experience. It's important to keep in mind that many others have gone before you (and surely many will come after you) in a helping mode. It's likely, too, that your host community is not a tabula rasa, (that is, a blank slate), and it may already have its own local approaches and successful interventions under way to address some of the global health problems you will encounter. Going to Africa with a "fix it" attitude is less helpful than approaching your experience there with humility, an openness to learning, and a willingness to listen closely. These three qualities will greatly increase your chances of creating an effective partnership with your counterparts and beneficiaries in Africa.

Enhance Your Communication Skills
Before you go, learn at least basic greetings in the main local language of your destination. In addition, learn when you should greet people casually (for instance, when interacting with your peers) and when you should be more formal (such as with your supervisors and elders). In many cultures, the proper way of greeting people differs according to age, relationship, and level of acquaintance, so that you should expect to offer different greetings to peers or children than to supervisors and elders. While it is not uncommon in the United States to refer to your friends' parents or some teachers by their first name, this would rarely be acceptable in Africa. An inherent respect for elders and those holding professional titles is more common in cultures outside of the United States; therefore, knowing the appropriate terms for respectful greetings and the use of formal titles is always recommended. In rural areas, this same approach should be applied to local leaders who may not have had formal education or acquired professional titles, but who hold a

prominent position in their communities. Greeting people appropriately, as well as your efforts to learn the local language, will show your
respect for the people with whom you are working. Learning as much
of the language as possible before you go will increase your effectiveness and self-sufficiency in your project role, and will open up opportunities for interacting with new colleagues and friends. If you can't take
a language course before you depart, consider options such as books,
audiotapes, and downloadable language tutorials to gain some facility
in the language.

Identify a Committed Advisor or Mentor

It's most useful to have an advisor or mentor with whom you communicate on a regular basis during your time abroad. A mentor might be
a faculty member at your academic institution, a staff member at the
agency sponsoring your trip, or a supervisor in your destination country. However, a mentor does not need to be physically present with you
in Africa. Communicating on a regular basis—weekly if possible—
can help you refine or alter your goals as needed, understand the experiences you are having, suggest new avenues and directions, and add
greatly to your learning.

Share Your Experiences

Sharing your experiences with others can help you reflect on what you
have seen and heard, informs others, and gives you useful ideas and
feedback about your work. One helpful technique is keeping a personal
journal or log. This will allow you to record experiences, keep track of
contacts, capture your perceptions, and document the plans and decisions that you make.

Many travelers recommend setting up a blog. This can afford you a
sizable following of readers and participants, and is particularly useful
if colleagues at home want to follow your travels and experiences in real
time. As another mode of communication, one student we know wrote
regularly during his travels to his clergyman at home, who then had the
letters published (with the writer's permission) in the congregational
newsletter, so an entire congregation "traveled" and learned along with
him. Remember that when using openly accessible tools, it's important
to consider the political and cultural sensitivity of all material that you
post. Humor, sarcasm, or criticism, no matter how mild, can be misin-

terpreted; when posting material publicly or sharing it with a wider audience, it is always best to err on the side of caution.

After you return home, giving talks at your academic institution, or to religious, cultural, or other interest groups on your campus or in the community are all good ways to share your experiences. Writing about your experiences for newsletters and your local newspaper, as well as in academic papers for courses, are all valuable ways to inform others and integrate your own experiences.

Many travelers bring a camera to capture their experience in photos. We encourage you to do so, but always be respectful of your subjects. Do keep in mind that many adults, especially those from more conservative cultures, may not appreciate having their photo taken, or may even be highly offended by being photographed. You should always ask permission (even if you do not speak the language, pointing to your camera can indicate your request) before clicking your photo. In busy outdoor scenes it is harder to obtain individual permissions, so it is best to ask a local co-worker or friend about the acceptability of taking photos in such settings. Children, on the other hand, almost always enjoy having their photo taken, especially if they can view the result on a digital camera screen immediately afterward. Often when children see a camera in your hands, they will ask you to take their picture. If you are not directly requested to take someone's picture, you should ask permission. If you plan to publish your photos in a print publication or show them in a presentation upon your return, especially if you might add a descriptive caption, we advise obtaining written permission from adults and verbal consent from children, with written permission from their parents or caretakers. Permission forms that you can adapt for this purpose may be available from your school's or sponsoring agency's newspaper or newsletter, or the public affairs or communications office.

Extend Your Learning

Continue to pursue some aspect of what you learned abroad through ongoing education after your return. Taking a course in some area related to your African experiences builds upon what you learned while there. For instance, after returning from a summer internship in a pediatric HIV clinic in Tanzania, one student we know discovered that her university offered Swahili. She continued courses in Swahili throughout college, increasing her language skills and facilitating her ability to communicate with friends and colleagues in Tanzania. She is keeping up the relationships she established there while she attends medical school, with the aim of going back to the country as a physician some day.

Build on Your Experiences

Proposing an ongoing project for the future is a viable way to extend your efforts in Africa. This might be a project you would carry out yourself (such as a research project, honors project, or thesis) or it might be work taken on by others who follow you. For example, several engineering undergraduates at our institution returned from a term in Tanzania having gathered sufficient community and scientific data to propose a project for building sustainable, self-composting latrines and improved cookstoves to reduce exposure to indoor air pollution. The project has been adopted by the student humanitarian engineering society on campus for implementation in several villages in western Tanzania. The students built working prototypes in their home academic setting, and in collaboration with the University of Dar es Salaam's College of Engineering and Technology, a second group of engineering students returned to implement the project in rural villages that requested this assistance. Because this is in a coffee-growing region of the country, the students successfully obtained funding for the project from a U.S. coffee company that imports coffee beans from that region of Tanzania and supports programs that improve the lives of coffee farmers, their families and their communities.[1]

Other travelers to Africa return home with an imperative to continue the work they started in some way. Several industrious travelers have put their efforts toward setting up their own NGOs. This requires a clear sense of purpose, careful legal guidance, and a willingness to do ongoing fundraising. This kind of initiative can extend the reach of your own work and maintain the professional relationships you formed while overseas. The sidebar, "Moved to Action," in the chapter on Tanzania, describes one such effort to establish an NGO and its early impact.

Returning Home

Returning home from an experience in Africa can entail a period of readaptation. How quickly and easily you readapt can be influenced by several things: the length of time you spend in Africa, the extent of interaction you have with the local population (versus with other foreigners), and your preparedness in advance for what you will find when you get there.

Individuals who spend several months or more in Africa sometimes find the readjustment to home takes longer and feels more intense than those who were there shorter periods of time. The lifestyle that you were accustomed to at home may suddenly seem superfluous and even overindulgent once you have seen people who are struggling with overwhelming poverty and harsh circumstances of disease. The location and kinds of activities you engage in while there can play a role as well. For instance, experiences that place you in remote areas with close daily interaction with the local population mean that you may well develop deep attachments to the people and the place. Separation when you depart can be intense.

In Africa, you will have gained a greater awareness of worldwide disparities in access to education, healthcare, and other basic services, which can sometimes lead to feeling discouraged and/or angry when you return home. Sometimes these emotions spur returnees to take action, locally or globally, to address some of the injustices they have witnessed. This can be a good time to seek out or reconnect with others who have traveled to the same or a similar destination or are from that country or region, to share your feelings and experiences. If your reaction to being home is one of prolonged sadness, a profound sense of loss, purposelessness, or trouble reengaging in your normal activities again, we strongly encourage you to seek mental health support. If you become physically ill within two months of returning home, or experience symptoms (such as fever or gastrointestinal discomfort) that do not seem to be resolving, you should seek medical attention.

Conclusion

Nothing can substitute for experience. The information in this book is designed to prepare you for your travel and work in Africa. Every traveler's experience is unique and intensely personal. We encourage you to:

Travel with an open mind. Always be in "learner mode," and consider your time in Africa an opportunity to see new and different approaches or ideas.

Be flexible. Things may not work out as you expect them to, but it
can be in these situations that some of the best cultural insights
can be learned.

Try to connect with the local population as much as possible. The
relationships you build will enhance your experience and give you
a greater understanding of the people and place you are visiting.

We hope your African experience is memorable and life changing.

NOTE

1. Dartmouth College Office of Public Affairs, "Dartmouth Receives Funding
for Global Health Project from Green Mountain Coffee," press release, July 23,
2009.

AIDS (see HIV/AIDS).

ART, or antiretroviral therapy (see also HIV/AIDS). The accepted multidrug therapy for treating HIV, ART consists of the use of at least three antiretroviral drugs to maximally suppress the HIV virus and halt progression of the disease. ART has produced huge reductions in death rates from HIV and is credited with shifting the status of HIV/AIDS from a fatal disease to a chronic one. Currently, an estimated thirty-three million people (thirty-one million adults and 2 million children) worldwide are living with HIV. Of these, over thirty million live in middle- and low-income countries. Two-thirds of all people infected with HIV reside in sub-Saharan Africa. Approximately five and one-quarter million (5.25 million) people had access to ART by the end of 2009, slightly more than half of all people in most urgent need of treatment. The World Health Organization sets ART treatment guidelines and provides support and guidance to countries in delivering therapy. To learn more, see http://www.who.int/hiv/topics/treatment/en/index.html.

CBOs, or community-based organizations. Nonprofit organizations that provide health or human services to meet the needs of local communities and populations (see also FBOs, NGOs).

Clinton Foundation. The foundation's global initiative has four major focus areas: education, energy and climate change, global health, and poverty elimination. President Bill Clinton established the Clinton HIV/AIDS Initiative (CHAI) in 2002, to close the gap in access to antiretroviral therapy (see ART) by negotiating lower prices and by working with governments to improve healthcare systems required to deliver ART. Since then, CHAI has expanded its scope, working to increase access to diagnostics and malaria medicines, and addressing issues related to the HIV/AIDS pandemic through (1) supporting governments to deliver HIV/AIDS services to underserved populations, such as children and those living in rural areas; (2) increasing countries' human resource capacity to deliver care and treatment; and (3) preventing the transmission of the disease from mothers to their children. To learn more, see http://www.clintonglobalinitiative.org.

DOTS. The internationally recommended strategy for tuberculosis control and the foundation for the current Stop TB Strategy, introduced in 2006, to reduce the global burden of the disease. Originally, the DOTS acronym stood for

Directly Observed Therapy—short course, describing two of the five essential components of the DOTS strategy. To bring attention back to all five components, the World Health Organization redefined DOTS as "the internationally agreed strategy for TB control." The five elements of the DOTS strategy are: (1) political commitment to increased and sustained financing for TB diagnosis and treatment; (2) case detection through quality-assured bacteriological tests; (3) standardized treatment, with supervision and patient support; (4) an effective drug supply and management system; (5) a monitoring and evaluation system and measurements of the program's impact. To learn more, see http://www.who.int/tb/dots/en/.

Endemic. The presence of a disease or infectious agent that is usual, constant, or highly prevalent within a geographic area or population. For example, malaria is endemic in many countries in Africa.

Epidemic. The occurrence of an illness that is clearly in excess of what is normally expected in a population or geographic area. The word is also used to describe sudden, unexpected outbreaks of disease.

External debt service. The total public and private debt of a country that is owed to outside creditors, and repayable in foreign currency, goods, or services. External debt can include money owed to banks, other governments, or international financial institutions such as the World Bank or the International Monetary Fund.

FBOs, or faith-based organizations. These organizations are religious in nature, as distinguished from governmental or public organizations, or those that are private and secular. The term came into common use following President George W. Bush's creation of the White House Faith-Based and Community Initiative, which seeks to assure that faith-based charities and organizations can compete with secular organizations for funding from the U.S. government to provide human services. Faith-based organizations have long played extensive roles in the provision of health and humanitarian aid services throughout the world, including in Africa.

Foreign direct investment. A company's physical investment in building a factory or providing machinery or equipment to build a business in another country, this may also include acquisition of a management interest in a company outside the home country, thus constructing a multinational corporation. Foreign direct investment plays a major role in the globalization of business.

Freedom House Index. This index is regarded as a measure of freedoms and civil liberties within a country. It is an aggregate measure that combines seven individual freedoms, including the right to: (1) participate freely in the political process; (2) vote freely in legitimate elections; (3) have accountable representatives; (4) exercise freedoms of expression and belief; (5) freely assemble and associate with others; (6) have access to an established and equitable system of rule and law; and (7) have social and economic freedoms, including equal access to economic opportunities and to hold private property. To learn more and read reports, see http://www.freedomhouse.org

GDP, or gross domestic product. The value of all goods and services produced within a country in a given year, the GDP is used as an aggregate statistic in a variety of indices, such as the United Nations Development Program's Human Development Index (see HDI).

Gini Index. A measure of the degree of inequality in distribution of income in a country, the index is commonly expressed on a scale of 0 to 100. In general, richer countries (as measured by high per capita GDP) tend to have intermediate Gini indices (under 40), while poorer countries have Gini indices with more variability, from low to very high (20s to 70s). Many European countries have Gini indices between 24 and 36; Japan's is 24.9, the United States' is 40.8, indicating greater inequality in income.

Global Fund to Fight AIDS, Tuberculosis and Malaria. This international fund was created in 2001 to increase resources to fight AIDS, TB, and malaria—the three most prevalent diseases in the world—which are estimated to kill over six million people each year. The fund solicits, manages, and disburses money to areas of greatest need. It operates solely as a financing mechanism; it does not implement or manage programs. The fund has disbursed $15.6 billion in grants to 140 countries. To learn more, see http://www.theglobalfund.org/en/.

HDI, or human development index. An aggregate index that combines three core elements of development: health, education, and the economy, the HDI is expressed as a value between 0 and 1. It takes into account life expectancy at birth (a measure of population health); adult literacy rate; combined gross enrollment ratios for primary, secondary, and tertiary schooling; and GDP per capita (PPP US$; see PPP). Developed by Mahbub ul Haq, a Pakistani economist, and Sir Richard Jolly, an English development economist, the HDI is thought to reflect human development on a broad level and is often used to rank countries. To learn more and find current statistics, see http://hdr.undp.org/en/. See also HPI, human development.

HIV/AIDS (see also ART; tuberculosis). Human immunodeficiency virus (HIV) is a retrovirus that infects cells of the human immune system, destroying them or impairing their function. In the early stages of infection, the person has no symptoms. Without treatment, the virus will multiply and, over time, cause the immune system to fail. As the infection progresses, the person becomes more susceptible to life-threatening opportunistic infections. The most advanced stage of HIV infection is acquired immunodeficiency syndrome (AIDS). It can take ten to fifteen years for an HIV-infected person to develop AIDS; multidrug therapy with antiretroviral medicines can slow the process significantly.

HIV is transmitted through unprotected sexual relations (particularly anal or vaginal intercourse), transfusion of contaminated blood, sharing of contaminated needles, and from a mother to her infant during pregnancy, childbirth, or breast-feeding. Source: http://www.who.int/topics/hiv_aids/en/.

As noted under Tuberculosis, HIV and tuberculosis are a deadly duo. Someone who is HIV-infected is much more likely to become sick with TB if they are newly infected with the TB bacilli or have a dormant TB infection. Once a person with HIV develops tuberculosis, their immune system is compromised further, allowing their HIV infection to progress. In this way, tuberculosis and HIV hasten each other's disease progression. Tuberculosis is the leading infectious cause of death among people who are HIV-infected. In Africa, HIV is the single most important factor contributing to the rise in TB over the last few decades. To learn more, see HIV/AIDS factsheets on a variety of topics and populations at http://www.cdc.gov/hiv/resources/factsheets/.

HPI, or Human Poverty Index. A measure of the paucity of choices available to individuals. Just as human development is the expansion of choices available to the individual, so human poverty is the reduction or denial of choices for a person to experience freedom, dignity, self-respect, and a decent standard of living. As an inverse measure of the elements reflected in the HDI, the HPI considers indicators of deprivation: a short life, lack of basic education, and lack of a decent standard of living. The HPI is derived separately for developing countries (HPI-1) and a select group of high-income countries (HPI-2) to better reflect socioeconomic differences and the widely different measures of deprivation within these country groupings. Components of the index include: (1) likeliness of death at a relatively early age, represented by the probability of not surviving to age forty in HPI-1 and to age sixty in HPI-2 countries; (2) the percentage of adults who are illiterate; (3) reflections of a decent standard of living, measured by the percentage of the population without access to safe water and the percentage of children underweight for age in HPI-1, and by the percentage of the population with incomes below the poverty level in HPI-2 countries. In addition, the HPI-2 index also includes the rate of long-term unemployment. The HPI in many African countries in this book is in the 50s to 70s; by comparison, the HPI for the United States is 15.4. To learn more, see http://hdr.undp.org/en/statistics/. See also HDI, human development.

Human development. The process of expanding the choices available to people, which gives them greater opportunities for income, employment, health care, and education.

Improved water source. Access to water considered safe—that is, provided through a household connection, public standpipe, borehole, protected well or spring, or rainwater collection. Improved water sources do not include vendors, tanker trucks, unprotected wells, unprotected springs, or bottled water. Access to an improved water source is commonly measured by the percentage of a population with daily access to at least twenty liters (5.3 gallons) of water from an improved source within 1 kilometer (0.62 mile, or slightly over a half mile) of the home.

Incidence. The occurrence of new cases of a disease in a population, incidence is a measure of the risk of getting a disease. It is usually expressed as a rate, which is calculated as the number of new cases of a disease in a population during a specified period of time (usually a year) divided by the size of the population. Incidence rates are usually expressed per 10,000 or 100,000 people.

Integrated Management of Childhood Illness (IMCI). This strategy was developed by WHO and UNICEF (see below for both) to reduce childhood morbidity and mortality in developing countries due to the five leading causes of death in childhood: malaria, diarrhea, measles, acute respiratory infections, and HIV/AIDS. The strategy promotes accurate identification of childhood illnesses, proper nutrition and immunization practices, the combined treatment of diseases in childhood, and rapid referral of severely ill children. There are three main components to the approach: "improving case management skills of health-care staff; improving overall health systems; [and] improving family and community health practices" (http://www.who.int/child_adolescent _health/topics/prevention_care/child/imci/en/index.html), such as appropriate care-seeking behavior and improved nutrition and preventive care. IMCI has been introduced in over seventy-five countries to date, and evaluations of the strategy suggest that it improves the quality of care, can reduce mortality in children under five, and "costs up to six times less per child . . . than current care" (ibid.).

Literacy rate. The percentage of the population aged fifteen and over who can read and write. Overall world literacy is estimated to be 82 percent. Throughout the world, higher literacy rates are associated with higher income, urban (as compared to rural) residence, and with positive health outcomes.

Malaria. This is a life-threatening disease caused by a parasite called *Plasmodium* which infects red blood cells. There are five types of human malaria—*P. falciparum*, *P. vivax*, *P. malariae*, *P. ovale* and *P. knowlesi*. The first two are the most common, and *P. falciparum* is by far the most deadly. Malaria is transmitted through the bite of an infected *Anopheles* mosquito. In humans, parasites grow and multiply in the liver and are released into the bloodstream where they infect red blood cells, causing them to burst as they release daughter parasites.

Symptoms of malaria usually begin 7 to 15 days after the infective mosquito bite. Fever, headache, chills, body aches and nausea/vomiting are the most common symptoms. Without treatment, malaria can progress quickly. Death occurs when the blood supply to vital organs has been compromised. Drug-resistant parasites are a problem in many endemic countries. Proven interventions to control malaria include: prompt and effective treatment with artemisinin-based combination therapies; use of insecticide-treated bed nets; and indoor spraying with insecticide to control the vector mosquitoes (http://www.who.int/topics/malaria/en/).

MDR TB, or multidrug-resistant tuberculosis. This is a specific form of drug-resistant TB that occurs when the bacteria are resistant to at least isoniazid and rifampicin, the two most powerful first-line drugs for treating the disease. MDR TB is much more challenging to treat than other forms of TB because most second-line medications are less effective, more toxic, and more expensive than first-line drugs.

Measles. An acute illness caused by a virus in the paramyxovirus family, measles virus normally grows in the cells that line the back of the throat and the lungs. Despite the availability of a safe and effective measles vaccine, the disease remains a leading cause of death for children under the age of five in many parts of the world. In 2008, there were an estimated 164,000 deaths worldwide from measles, mostly among young children. Measles is extremely contagious, so that almost all children who are not immune will develop the disease if exposed to the virus. The virus is spread by coughing and sneezing, or by close personal contact. Measles can cause severe illness or death in young children, particularly those who are poorly nourished, do not receive sufficient vitamin A, or those whose immune systems have been weakened by HIV/AIDS or other diseases. Children usually do not die directly of measles, but from its complications, which can include blindness, encephalitis (a dangerous infection of the brain causing inflammation), severe diarrhea (leading to dehydration), and severe respiratory infections such as pneumonia, which is the most common cause of death associated with measles. To learn more, see http://www.who.int/mediacentre/factsheets/fs286/en/.

Neonatal Tetanus. In many countries, deliveries take place in unhygienic circumstances, posing a serious risk for the mother and child to get infected by tetanus (see also Tetanus). Non-sterile delivery, contamination of the umbilical cord by cutting with a non-sterile instrument, or local customs of treating the cord stump with dirt or animal dung can introduce tetanus. Once infected, mortality rates are extremely high, especially in areas where appropriate medical care is not available. However, these deaths can easily be prevented by either clean, safe delivery practices and/or by immunizing the mothers. Approximately 8% of all neonatal deaths are due to neonatal tetanus. Cases occur mostly in Africa and Southeast Asia. Worldwide, 69 percent of pregnant women are protected against tetanus. (Source: http://www.who.int/immunization_monitoring/diseases/MNTE_initiative/en/index.html.)

NGOs. Nongovernmental organizations include a wide variety of agencies, organizations, and foundations that address a broad range of issues in all parts of the world. Also called private voluntary organizations, civil societies, or citizen associations, the term "NGO" is increasingly preferred to distinguish these agencies from governmental agencies. NGOs usually have little power in international decision making, but they have been successful in promoting human rights and social justice; environmental agreements; women's rights; arms control and disarmament measures; and improved rights and protections for children, the disabled, the poor, and indigenous peoples. You may hear NGOs referred to as "non-state actors," suggesting their increasing influence in the international policy arena where previously only governments, or states, played a significant role. There are an estimated 25,000 international NGOs with programs or affiliates worldwide. NGOs distinguish themselves from other nonprofit organizations by their advocacy role. Former UN Secretary General Kofi Annan called NGOs "the conscience of humanity." (Source: Koffi Annan, quoted in *The UN Security Council: from the Cold War to the 21st Century*, ed. David M. Malone, p. 374 [Boulder: Lynne-Rienner Publishers, 2004].)

Official development assistance (ODA). Development assistance from the Organization for Economic Cooperation and Development (OECD) nations to developing countries and multilateral organizations, the objective of this assistance is to promote economic development in less developed countries.

Pandemic. An epidemic of disease that is worldwide, crossing national borders.

PEPFAR, or the President's Emergency Plan for AIDS Relief. The plan was announced by President George W. Bush in his 2003 State of the Union address. PEPFAR initially dedicated $15 billion over five years to combating HIV internationally. The plan's five-year global strategy guides its work with international, national, and local organizations in programs aimed at prevention, treatment, and health care. PEPFAR was reauthorized by Congress in 2008 to provide $48 million through 2013. The aspect of the plan that has received the most criticism is its strategy to prevent new HIV infection among young people. With the knowledge that in some areas of Africa one of every three-four new infections occurs among people under twenty-five, and primarily among young women, the plan promotes a strategy of "ABC" prevention messages: "A" promotes sexual abstinence, or delaying the start of sexual activity for young people; "B" stresses being faithful to one partner, or reducing the number of sexual partners; and "C" emphasizes correct and consistent condom use, where appropriate. To learn more, see http://www.pepfar.gov.

PPP, or Purchasing Power Parity. A measure that equalizes the purchasing power of different currencies in their home countries, it thereby controls for the value of these currencies. PPP is the monetary value of basic goods that are bought in a given country by using the money that the country produces.

President's Malaria Initiative (PMI). Initiated by President George W. Bush in June 2005, the PMI increased U.S. funding of malaria programs by $1.2 billion over five years, with the aim of reducing malaria deaths by 50 percent in fifteen African countries. The legislation reauthorizing PEPFAR (see above) allocated $5 billion for the PMI. Funding supports four effective prevention strategies: indoor spraying of homes with insecticides, insecticide-treated mosquito nets, antimalarial drugs, and treatment to prevent malaria in pregnant women. The initiative is led by USAID (see below), in conjunction with the Centers for Disease Control and Prevention, the Department of State, and the White House, and it works with national malaria control programs and international partners. To learn more, see http://www.fightingmalaria.gov/.

Prevalence. The number of cases of a disease that exist at a point in time or over a period of time. Prevalence is expressed as a rate, which is calculated as the number of cases of a disease present in a population at a specified period of time divided by the number of people at risk of having the disease. For example, in several countries in sub-Saharan Africa, the prevalence of HIV in adults has exceeded 15 percent (or 15,000 per 100,000 population). Unlike incidence, which is a measure of risk, prevalence is a measure of the burden of disease in a society.

Schistosomiasis, or bilharzia. This is a parasitic disease caused by trematode flatworms called Schistosoma. In some parts of the world, including many areas in Africa, freshwater snails carry the larvae of the parasites, releasing them into the water, where the larvae can easily penetrate the skin of people in the water and go undetected. Once in the human body, the larvae develop into adult schistosomes, which live in blood vessels. Eggs released by female schistosomes can lodge in body tissues, causing an immune reaction. The disease can take several forms in humans, for instance, in urinary schistosomiasis, there is progressive damage to the bladder, ureters and kidneys. In intestinal schistosomiasis, there is progressive enlargement of the liver and spleen, intestinal damage, and hypertension of the abdominal blood vessels. Control methods for schistosomiasis include drug treatment of the disease, snail control, improved sanitation and health education. Schistosomiasis is the reason you are cautioned against swimming in fresh water (rivers, streams and lakes) in Africa. To learn more, see http://www.who.int/topics/schistosomiasis/en/.

Tetanus. A vaccine-preventable, non-communicable disease, it is acquired through environmental exposure to the spores of the bacterium Clostridium tetani, which produce a neurotoxin. The spores are widespread in the environment. The disease is caused by the action of the neurotoxin, produced by the bacteria when they grow in the absence of oxygen, for example, in dirty wounds or in the umbilical cord if it is cut with a non-sterile instrument. Tetanus is characterized by muscle spasms, initially in the jaw. As the disease progresses, mild stimuli may trigger generalized tetanic seizure-like activity, which contributes to serious complications and eventual death unless supportive treatment is given.

Tetanus can be prevented by the administration of tetanus toxoid, which induces specific antitoxins. To prevent maternal and neonatal tetanus, tetanus toxoid needs to be given to the mother before or during pregnancy, and clean delivery and umbilical cord care needs to be ensured. (Source: http://www.who.int/topics/tetanus/en/.)

Tuberculosis (TB). An infectious bacterial disease caused by *Mycobacterium tu-berculosis*, it most commonly affects the lungs. Transmission occurs when an infected person sneezes, coughs, spits or sings and releases infectious respiratory droplets into the air and an uninfected person inhales them. The TB bacilli travel to the terminal airways of the lung where they are walled off by a healthy immune system. In most healthy people, the TB bacilli will remain walled off and in a dormant state, called latent TB infection, for the rest of their life. In a minority, the bacilli will multiple and cause a person to become sick with TB disease. When someone's immune system is weakened, the chances of becoming sick are greater. Only people who are sick with TB in their lungs are contagious.

The main symptoms of TB disease of the lung are cough, sometimes with bloody sputum, fever, weight loss, and night sweats. In the vast majority of patients, tuberculosis can be cured with a six-month course of antibiotics. In most countries, treatment is done primarily on an outpatient basis, reserving hospitalization only for the sickest who may need intravenous medicines or fluids. To learn more, see http://www.who.int/topics/tuberculosis/en/.

As noted under HIV/AIDS, HIV and tuberculosis are a deadly duo. Someone who is HIV-infected is much more likely to become sick with TB if they are newly infected with the TB bacilli or have a dormant TB infection. Once a person with HIV develops tuberculosis, their immune system is compromised further, allowing their HIV infection to progress. In this way, tuberculosis and HIV hasten each other's progression. Tuberculosis is the leading infectious cause of death among people who are HIV-infected. In Africa, HIV is the single most important factor contributing to the rise in TB over the last few decades. To learn more, see http://www.cdc.gov/hiv/resources/factsheets for information on HIV and TB co-infection.

UNAIDS, or the Joint United Nations Programme on HIV/AIDS. This agency brought together ten UN-related organizations to mount an expanded global response to AIDS. The aims of UNAIDS are to help countries prevent new HIV infections, care for people living with HIV, and mitigate the impact of the epidemic. UNAIDS is currently working in more than eighty countries. To learn more, see http://www.unaids.org/en/.

UNICEF, or the United Nations Children's Fund. Under a mandate from the UN and guided by the UN Convention on the Rights of the Child, UNICEF advocates for protection of children worldwide, believing that "nurturing and caring for children are the cornerstones of human progress" (http://www.unicef.org/about/who/index.html). Its activities aim to overcome the obstacles that children face, including poverty, violence, disease and discrimination. UNICEF programs target child survival, nutrition, environmental interventions, basic education, gender equity, pediatric treatment of HIV/AIDS, and protection of children from violence, exploitation, and abuse. Above all, UNICEF programs emphasize low-cost, low-technology, high-impact interventions such as vaccines, antibiotics, micronutrient supplements, insecticide-treated bed nets, improved breast-feeding practices, and adoption of safe hygiene practices that can prevent unnecessary maternal and child deaths. The agency monitors and provides statistics on the status of women and children worldwide. To learn more, see http://www.unicef.org/.

USAID, or the U.S. Agency for International Development. A federal agency created in 1961, USAID provides economic and humanitarian assistance in five regions of the world: sub-Saharan Africa, Asia, Latin America and the Caribbean, Europe and Eurasia, and the Middle East. The agency partners with voluntary organizations, local organizations, universities, American businesses, international agencies, and foreign governments. By supporting economic development, agriculture and trade, global health, democracy, conflict prevention, and humanitarian assistance in foreign countries the agency fosters economic growth, along with U.S. foreign policy objectives internationally. USAID spends less than half of 1 percent of the U.S. federal budget each year toward these aims. To learn more see: http://www.usaid.gov/.

WHO. The World Health Organization is the United Nations' authority on global health. It sets standards, shapes policies, provides technical support to countries on health issues, and monitors health trends around the world. Conceived in the discussions that formed the United Nations in 1945, WHO became a reality on 7 April 1948, a date now celebrated as World Health Day. To learn more, see http://www.who.int/en/.

XDR TB, or extensively drug-resistant tuberculosis. A form of MDR TB (see also MDR TB) that is resistant not only to first-line drug treatment but also to certain second-line medications, specifically any one of the drugs in the fluoroquinolone family and to at least one of three injectable second-line drugs (amikacin, capreomycin, or kanamycin). Treatment outcomes for patients with XDR TB are even worse than for those with MDR TB. XDR TB was first widely publicized following reports of a 2006 outbreak in KwaZulu-Natal, South Africa (see the South Africa chapter for more details). XDR TB can have a very high mortality rate in patients co-infected with HIV.

LISA V. ADAMS, M.D., is an assistant professor in the Department of Medicine, Section of Infectious Disease and International Health, Dartmouth Medical School. She has been working in domestic and international TB control for over fifteen years, and has provided technical assistance to national TB programs, led assessment missions for new TB collaborative projects, and developed indicators for monitoring and evaluating TB control programs in Eastern Europe, Central Asia and sub-Saharan Africa. At Dartmouth, she teaches courses on global health and directs Dartmouth's Global Health Initiative at the Dickey Center for International Understanding, through which she develops and oversees several cross-cutting global health programs involving faculty and students. She is also involved in the DarDar Programs, Dartmouth's tuberculosis and HIV/AIDS clinical research and care programs conducted in collaboration with Muhimbili University of Health and Allied Sciences in Dar es Salaam, Tanzania.

PALAV BABARIA, M.D., was a fourth year medical student at Yale University at the time she contributed to this book. As an undergraduate at Harvard University she majored in South Asian Studies, focusing on issues of gender-based violence in immigrant and refugee populations. After college, she volunteered for several NGOs working with underprivileged children in Mumbai, India. During medical school, she lived in Tugela Ferry, South Africa from 2007–2008 as an International Doris Duke Clinical Research Fellow, examining risk factors for delayed diagnosis among TB-HIV co-infected individuals, and continues to work with the Tugela Ferry Care and Research Collaboration (TF CaRes) on their active TB case detection studies. She is interested in working with marginalized populations domestically and internationally, with a special interest in HIV and gender-based violence.

STEPHANIE WILLMAN BORDAT, J.D., has been director of the Morocco field office for the international NGO Global Rights since 2000. In 2003, she expanded it into a Maghreb-wide regional program. Her work involves the design and implementation of projects in collaboration with local NGOs and lawyers in diverse areas across Morocco, Algeria and Tunisia to enhance knowledge of legal and human rights among illiterate and semi-literate women; conducting, monitoring and documenting women's rights violations in the formal justice system; advocating for legislation in the area of violence against women;

promoting the use of the marriage contract as a tool to protect women's rights; and encouraging strategic litigation in front of domestic courts. Prior to joining Global Rights, she worked with NGOs in Pakistan, Egypt and the Netherlands, conducting legal research on women's human rights issues including the status of migrant sex workers, violence against women, such as honour killings, and country strategies to meet their obligations under international human rights conventions. She was a Fulbright Scholar at the Université Mohammed V in Rabat, Morocco, where she studied Islamic Family Law, Personal Status Codes, and the status of women in Morocco. She first came to Morocco as a Peace Corps volunteer. She holds law degrees with honors from both Columbia Law School in New York and the Université Paris I-Sorbonne in France.

NAMEETA M. DOOKERAN, M.D., M.SC., is director of the Global Health Rotation for the Internal Medicine Residency Program of Brigham and Women's Hospital, Boston, and an associate physician in the hospital's Hospitalist Service. She has been involved in a variety of global health projects, first in India and Nepal as a medical student in 2000, and then in Ghana in 2004 during her medical residency, where she worked in Ghana's first HIV clinic. She is a member of the board of the Boston-based Foundation for African Relief, through which she first went to Ghana. Her interests include global health residency curriculum development and program development to increase health care delivery in underserved populations.

THOMAS EISELE, M.P.H., PH.D., is an assistant professor in the Department of International Health and Development at the Tulane School of Public Health and Tropical Medicine. With expertise in epidemiology, community intervention strategies for controlling malaria, monitoring and evaluation, and survey sampling methodology, his research focuses on the use of epidemiologic methods for evaluating community public health interventions in developing country settings. His primary interests in malaria research include: measuring malaria transmission; evaluating community-based malaria control programs; assessing social determinants of malaria control intervention uptake and adherence; and investigating the relationship between transmission pressure and child mortality.

NEEL R. GANDHI, M.D., is a physician-epidemiologist who has been engaged in clinical research in tuberculosis and HIV co-infection since 1998. Dr. Gandhi is a founding member and a principal investigator in the Tugela Ferry Care and Research (TF CaRes) Collaboration, an international group of healthcare professionals focusing on epidemiological and operational research studies to improve care for HIV and TB in rural, resource-limited settings. In November 2006, he was the lead author on a study describing high rates of mortality in patients with extensively drug-resistant tuberculosis and HIV co-infection. This study has been credited for uncovering a rapidly expanding multidrug-resistant (MDR) TB and XDR TB epidemic in South Africa. Currently, his efforts focus on expanding TB/HIV integration activities in rural South Africa; elucidating risk factors for and combating MDR and XDR TB and HIV in South Africa; and creating a community-based treatment program for MDR TB in HIV co-infected patients. He is an assistant professor of medicine and epidemiology at Albert Einstein College of Medicine and Montefiore Medical Center, Bronx, New York.

LAURA J. HAAS, M.B.A., PH.D., is the director of Tulane University's Rwanda Country Office, a research associate professor in the Payson Center for International Development and Technology Transfer at Tulane, and a visiting lecturer at the National University of Rwanda's School of Public Health. She oversees Tulane's portfolio of projects in Rwanda and since 2002, has provided direct support to the institutional development efforts at the School of Public Health in Rwanda. She also supports the regional Health Alliance initiative, a network of seven institutions of higher learning in public health in East and Central Africa. Dr. Haas has worked with health systems throughout Africa, including in the Democratic Republic of the Congo, Kenya, Rwanda, Uganda, Cameroon, Côte d'Ivoire, and Senegal among others. Her areas of expertise include institutional capacity development; program development and management; operations research, curriculum design and implementation of graduate level training programs in Africa; human resources for health planning, management, and development; and improved adult pedagogy through instructional design technology and distance education.

ACHILLES KATAMBA, M.B.CH.B., D.C.H., PH.D., is a lecturer in the Clinical Epidemiology and Biostatistics Unit, Department of Medicine, School of Medicine, College of Health Sciences, Makerere University, Uganda. He teaches epidemiology and research methodology to graduate and undergraduate students and health services research to graduate students in the Master of Health Services degree program. His research interests include tuberculosis, clinical decision-making, cost-effectiveness, and operations research. Dr. Katamba is a faculty member on the Joint Clinical Research Center/Case Western Reserve University's Comprehensive International Clinical Operational and Health Services Training Grant for AIDS and TB.

SAIDA KOUZZI, J.D., is an attorney and women's rights activist from Ouezzane, Morocco. She is the Regional Legal Officer for the Maghreb Regional Office of Global Rights. She develops and conducts trainings on women's human rights issues and institutional development strategies; coordinates action-research projects; and designs and carries out advocacy campaigns. She co-authors the Maghreb Regional Office Arabic language publications, which include: "Making Human Rights Real: A Legal Literacy Program for Women in Morocco," "Resource Book on Empowering Girls and Young Women at Risk in Morocco," "Promoting Women's Rights in the Maghreb through Strategic Use of the Marriage Contract," "A Practical Guide for NGOs to implement and conduct

Court Accompaniment for Women," "The Young Women Activist's Guide to Network-Building," and "Promoting Women's Rights in the Maghreb: A Resource Guide for Litigating International Law in Domestic Courts." She advocated on behalf of Moroccan women during several sessions of the U.N. Human Rights Commission in Geneva, where she also co-led a delegation for the Global Rights Advocacy Bridge Program. She earned her law degree from Mohammed V University in Rabat.

HENRY LUZZE, M.B.CH.B., M.S., is director of research coordination at the Uganda–Case Western Reserve University Research Collaboration, Mulago Hospital Complex, in Uganda.

NANCY B. MOCK, Dr.P.H., is the interim executive director of the Newcomb College Center for Research on Women and an associate professor of international health and development at Tulane University. She has over thirty years of experience in humanitarian and development work, concentrating on the problems of higher education in development, food security and health sector development, and has worked in more than thirty countries in Africa, Asia, Latin America and Eastern Europe. Since 2000, she has worked intensively with the government of Rwanda to strengthen local leadership and capacity of public health institutions, and was instrumental in the establishment of the National University of Rwanda's School of Public Health. In addition to Rwanda, she has helped to establish university-based schools or units of public health in Senegal, the Democratic Republic of Congo, Uganda and Vietnam. Dr. Mock leads Tulane University's component of the Leadership Initiative for Public Health in East Africa, an initiative bringing together seven schools and departments of public health in the East and Central African region.

BARUDI MOSIMANEOTSILE, M.P.H., B.Ed., is a nurse epidemiologist at the Botswana-USA (BOTUSA) partnership TB/HIV unit in Botswana. She earned an MPH in epidemiology from the University of Hawaii School of Public Health in 1999, and a nursing degree from University of Botswana in 1994. She has more than ten years of experience working in the field of TB/HIV, as a public health senior lecturer at the Institute of Health Sciences in Botswana, and as a researcher coordinating various BOTUSA research projects. For the past seven years at BOTUSA, she has dedicated her efforts to the implementation and coordination of TB/HIV projects, mainly in the area of Isoniazid TB preventive therapy. Her work has included implementation and coordination of the government Isoniazid preventive therapy pilot program, which has now been implemented nationwide. Currently she is a study coordinator for the ongoing clinical trial of different treatment regimens for latent TB in people living with HIV.

HELGA NABURI, M.D., M.P.H., is a lecturer in the Department of Pediatrics at Muhimbili University of Health and Allied Sciences, in Dar es Salaam, Tanzania. She is also the clinical director of the DarDar Pediatric Program in Dar es

Salaam, a care and treatment center for HIV-infected youth, jointly administered by Muhimbili University of Health and Allied Sciences and Dartmouth Medical School. In 2007–08 she was a Fogarty Fellow at Dartmouth College in the Fogarty Center-sponsored AIDS International Training and Research Program, and earned a Master of Public Health degree from The Dartmouth Institute for Clinical Practice and Health Policy.

JAMES OLOYA, D.V.M., PH.D., is an assistant professor of epidemiology in the Department of Epidemiology and Biostatistics, University of Georgia College of Public Health. Trained in veterinary medicine, he has a special interest in microbial food safety and antimicrobial drug resistance of food-borne zoonoses. He has studied the epidemiology of bovine and environmental mycobacteria at the domestic animal-human interface in the pastoral areas of Uganda. Currently he teaches food safety and veterinary epidemiology at the University of Georgia Colleges of Public Health and of Veterinary Medicine.

JOYCE A. SACKEY, M.D., is dean for multicultural affairs and global health programs at Tufts University School of Medicine. Prior to assuming her position at Tufts in March 2009, she was a primary care physician at Beth Israel Deaconess Medical Center (BIDMC), Boston, and associate master for the Oliver Wendell Holmes Society at Harvard Medical School where she served on the faculty. She is co-founder of the Foundation for African Relief, a Massachusetts-based non-profit organization, and directs the BIDMC-based AIDS Collaborative Project and its Visiting Scholar's Exchange Program, a program contributing to the fight against AIDS in Ghana and Sudan by training African physicians to provide clinical care to people living with HIV/AIDS. Through the AIDS Collaborative Project, she encourages physicians both locally and abroad to address health care disparities by expanding their clinical skills to include specific skills in cultural competency. She mentors and advises medical students and residents interested in international health, many of whom have undertaken international projects in Ghana, Liberia and Uganda. She was awarded the Gold Foundation Award for Humanism in Medicine from Harvard Medical School (2005) and Dartmouth College's Martin Luther King Social Justice Award (2004) in recognition of her work in addressing training and treatment gaps in global HIV/AIDS.

STELLA SAFO, B.A., was a third-year medical student at Harvard Medical School when she contributed to this book. She is a graduate of Harvard College with a B.A. in History of Science and African American studies. A child of Ghanaian natives, she was born in Nigeria. Her interests in HIV/AIDS treatment and prevention programs in Ghana have led her to return to there often. She has conducted field research on HIV stigmatization in Ghana, consulted for the national support group for HIV positive Ghanaians, and overseen prevention programs at local high schools. Her goal is to become a primary care physician with a particular focus on women's health and HIV/AIDS.

She will shortly obtain an MPH degree from the Harvard School of Public Health's international track as a Zuckerman fellow, in addition to her medical degree.

MICHELLE SCOTT, B.A., was a medical student at Harvard Medical School at the time she contributed to this book. Her interest in international public health began as an undergraduate at Stanford University where she majored in Human Biology with a focus on international health. After graduating Stanford she joined the Peace Corps and worked in Cote d'Ivoire and Madagascar as a public health volunteer and collaborated with community health workers and local health clinics to develop educational programs focusing on maternal and infant health, adolescent reproductive health, and HIV/AIDS. During medical school Michelle worked on projects developing TB and HIV education programs at a community center in Namibia, and in 2007–08 she worked in the community based treatment program for MDR TB patients at the Tugela Ferry Care and Research (TF CaRes) Collaboration in Tugela Ferry, South Africa.

LAUREL A. SPIELBERG, M.A., M.P.H., Dr.P.H., is both an epidemiologist and a social worker, with particular interests in the health of women and children. She is currently a public health consultant, and develops educational modules focused on global maternal and child health and public health issues. She has spent over thirty-five years in a wide variety of positions in public health and social work in the US and Canada, both as faculty at schools of public health and as an epidemiologist for city, county, and provincial (Canadian) health departments. Her areas of expertise are reproductive health, maternal and child health, community-based epidemiology, the impacts of social and environmental factors on health, and the planning and evaluation of health and social service programs.

ELIZABETH A. TALBOT, M.D., is an associate professor of medicine at Dartmouth Medical School and serves as Deputy State Epidemiologist and TB Medical Advisor for the New Hampshire Department of Health and Human Services. She is a medical scientist for the Foundation for Innovative New Diagnostics in Geneva. Dr. Talbot has extensive experience in international health, and received education in tropical medicine at the London School of Hygiene and Tropical Medicine. She is a Diplomate in both Tropical and Travel Medicine. During medical residency at Duke University Medical Center, she trained in Brazil, practicing tertiary care tropical medicine and conducting research in the transmission of multidrug-resistant tuberculosis. She had comprehensive training in TB epidemiology, diagnosis, treatment and control at National Jewish Medical Center in Denver, and training in epidemiology and public health with the Epidemic Intelligence Service of the Centers for Disease Control and Prevention (CDC), working for five years in the field station in Botswana (2 as an EIS officer, 3 as Associate Director for TB/HIV Research). While in Botswana, Dr. Talbot represented the CDC in international venues such as the

World Health Organization's TB/HIV Working Group, and was primary mentor to many local professional staff and US medical students.

RICHARD WADDELL, D.Sc., is a research assistant professor of medicine in the Section of Infectious Disease and International Health at Dartmouth Medical School. He also directs the AIDS Education and Training Center, in New Hampshire, and is a program consultant for the Global Health Initiative at Dartmouth's Dickey Center for International Understanding. He has over twenty years of experience in epidemiologic and clinical research on HIV and TB in international settings, including the Caribbean, Central America, Europe, and the Democratic Republic of Congo, Kenya, Zambia, and Tanzania in sub-Saharan Africa. He mentors undergraduate and graduate students at Dartmouth, and works directly with international fellows in the Fogarty Center-funded AIDS International Training and Research Program focusing on HIV and TB. Dr. Waddell's training is in epidemiology and health services research.

CLAIRE WAGNER, B.A., received her undergraduate degree in anthropology from Dartmouth College in 2010. She served as intern for the Global Health Initiative of Dartmouth's Dickey Center for International Understanding at the time she contributed to this book. Claire has worked in Costa Rica as a teacher, and in Mali as a project coordinator and instructor of outdoor emergency medicine. She served as the Global Health Intern for Children's Hospital Boston's International Health Services Department, and on a research team in Mali with Massachusetts General Hospital's Division of Global Health and Human Rights. She has spoken on several panels, including Dartmouth Medical School's Great Issues in Medicine and Global Health Lecture Series, and the Center for Strategic and International Studies' meeting on The Future of Global Health. Based on her research in Tanzania, she wrote her undergraduate thesis, "Into the Street: Children's agency, adaptation and survival in Dar es Salaam, Tanzania." Currently, she works for Harvard Medical School's Department of Global Health and Social Medicine as the Research Assistant to the Permanent Secretary of the Ministry of Health of Rwanda.

CHARLES WELLS, M.D., currently serves as medical director for the Tuberculosis Products Unit at Otsuka Pharmaceutical Development and Commercialization. From January 2001 to May 2007, he served as chief of the International Research and Programs Branch within the Division of Tuberculosis Elimination at the Centers for Disease Control and Prevention (CDC). The branch he led at the CDC has been a leading technical group for epidemiologic, clinical, and diagnostics research on TB and for providing direct technical assistance internationally for implementation and scale up of programs for TB, TB/HIV (within PEPFAR), and multidrug-resistant (MDR) TB. Board Certified in both internal medicine and infectious disease, he began his research efforts in tuberculosis in 1995, upon joining the Epidemiology Intelligence Service (EIS) at

CDC, and has remained working in the field since that time. While at CDC, his group successfully launched a 2000 patient clinical trial in Botswana in 2004, evaluating the optimal duration for isoniazid preventive therapy for persons living with HIV in TB endemic settings. During his fourteen years of working in TB, TB/HIV, and multidrug (MDR) resistant TB, he has worked in many countries including Vietnam, Cambodia, Thailand, Philippines, India, Russia, the Baltic countries, South Africa, Botswana, Ethiopia, Brazil, and Mexico, among others.

CHRISTOPHER C. WHALEN, M.D., M.S., is a professor of epidemiology in the Department of Epidemiology and Biostatistics at the University of Georgia College of Public Health. He received his medical and epidemiologic degrees from Case Western Reserve University, where he was a faculty member for eighteen years. He first began working in Uganda in 1990, with a focus on the prevention and treatment of tuberculosis in HIV-infected patients. He expanded the scope of his work in 1995 to examine the transmission dynamics of TB in African households. He has been the director of the AIDS International Training and Research Program and the International Clinical, Operational, and Health Services Research Award, through which he has directed the training of over fifty Ugandan graduate students.

Italicized page numbers indicate entries in the country-data tables that appear at the end of chapters.

ABC approach to HIV prevention, 205
abortion, 103–5
African Comprehensive HIV/AIDS Partners (ACHAP), 50
African history, 6–7
African Medical and Research Foundation, 211–12
African National Congress (ANC), 160–61, 163, 171
Afrikaner, 158
Afrikaner National Party, 159, 160
AIDS. *See* HIV/AIDS
Amin, Idi, 197, 228
antiretroviral therapy (ART): in Botswana, 48, 50, 51; in Ghana, 75, 76, 80–81; in Rwanda, 130, 132, 134, 139; in South Africa, 167, 173–75, 177; in Tanzania, 203–5, 208, 212; in Uganda, 236–38, 244, 245
antimalarial drugs or treatment; in Rwanda, 132, 133; in Tanzania, 209; for traveler, 31; in Uganda, 240. *See also* artemisinin-based combination therapy
apartheid, 156–57, 179, 182; health-care system under, 167–68; 174; by law, 159–60; the mines and,165–66; political resistance to, 160–61; post-apartheid, 161–62, 164
artemisinin-based combination therapy: in Ghana, 76–77; in

Tanzania, 209. *See also* antimalarial drugs or treatment
Asante tribe, 64–65

Baganda, 248
Bantu, 196, 228; Bantu laws, 159, 164; Bantu state, 167
Batswana, 43, 44, 61n6
Baylor College of Medicine, 46
bed nets. *See* insecticide-treated bed nets
Bibi Jann School, 206–7
bilharzia. *See* schistosomiasis
Bill and Melinda Gates Foundation; in Botswana, 50; Gates Grand Challenges in Global Health, 17–18
blog, 38, 258
Boer, 43, 158
Botswana Christian ADIS Intervention Program (BOCAIP), 50–51
BOTUSA (Botswana-USA), 48, 50–51
breast-feeding, 139, 204, 210–11
Bristol Myers Squibb Foundation, 50–51
Bushmen, 51–52

cardiovascular disease, 171, 178–79
CDC. *See* Centers for Disease Control and Prevention
Centers for Disease Control and Prevention (CDC): in Botswana, 48,

in Rwanda, 122, 124, 127, 128; in Uganda, 243

miners, 165–67

mother-to-child-transmission of HIV (MTCT). See Prevention of mother-to-child transmission (PMTCT)

Muhimbili University of Health and Allied Sciences (MUHAS), 201, 213

multidrug-resistant tuberculosis (MDR TB): in Botswana, 50, *59*; in Ghana, *86*; in the Maghreb, *114*; in Rwanda, 137, *148*; in South Africa, 156, 175, 177–78, *187*; in Tanzania, 208, *221*; in Uganda, 238, 252

Muslims: in Ghana, 67; in the Maghreb, 93; in South Africa, 163; in Tanzania, 197. *See also* Islam

national health insurance. *See* health insurance

National University of Rwanda, 130, 141, 142

neonatal tetanus. *See* tetanus

Noguchi Memorial Institute for Medical Research, 79

nongovernmental organizations (NGOs), 260; in Botswana, 47, 48, 50; in Ghana, 76, 78, 80; in the Maghreb, 96, 97, 104, 106, 107–8, 108–10; NGO Code, 20n7; in Rwanda, 130, 140, 142; in South Africa, 174, 175, 176; in Tanzania, 198, 199, 206–7, 212, 213; in Uganda, 235, 243, 248

Nyerere, Julius, 195–96, 197

obesity, 178–79

official development assistance: Botswana, *57*; Ghana, *84*; the Maghreb, *112*; Rwanda, *146*; South Africa, *185*; Tanzania, *219*; Uganda, *250*

orphan care: in South Africa, 176; in Tanzania, 213

orphans: in Botwana, 47; in Rwanda, 134, 135–37; in Tanzania, 202, 205, 206–7, 224–25n32; in Uganda, 233, 234

packing list, 38–39

pandemic, 6

passport information, 29–30

Peace Corps: in Ghana, 63; in Morocco, 110; in Tanzania, 213

photography guidance for travelers, 259

Plasmodium falciparum, 76, 132, 239–40

poverty: in Ghana, 68; link to health, 11; millennium development goal related to, 18, 19; in Rwanda, 124, 126, 135; in South Africa, 164, 171, 173; in Tanzania, 196, 206; in Uganda, 229, 238, 241

President's Emergency Plan for AIDS Relief (PEPFAR): in Botswana, 51; in Rwanda, 134; in Tanzania, 203, 212–13, 215; in Uganda, 237

President's Malaria Initiative (PMI): in Rwanda, 133; in Tanzania, 212

prevention of mother-to-child transmission (PMTCT): in Ghana, 76, 79; in Rwanda, 134; in South Africa, 173, 174, 175; in Tanzania, 199, 204–5, 212; in Uganda, 237, 246

private healthcare or insurance: in Botswana, 47; in Ghana, 71; in South Africa, 168, 171; in Uganda, 232

Purchasing Power Parity (PPP): Botswana, *57*, *58*; Ghana, *84*, *86*; the Maghreb, *112*, *114*; Rwanda, *146*, *148*; South Africa, *185*, *187*; Tanzania, *219*, *221*; Uganda, *250*, *252* rabies, 241, 242

Rakai Health Sciences Program, 246

rape. *See* violence against women

refugees: Rwandan, 123, 125; in Tanzania, 197

religions: Botswana, *56*; Ghana, *83*; the Maghreb, *111*; Rwanda, *145*; South Africa, *184*; Tanzania, *218*; Uganda, *249*. *See also* Islam; Muslims

religious extremism, 95–96

reproductive health. *See* family planning

returning home, re-adaptation, 260–61

Roll Back Malaria Campaign, 240

safety: and security, 35; traffic-related, 35–36, 77–78, 180

Sahara Desert, 92, 95

SALAMA Tanzania, 206–7

schistosomiasis, 31

Sector Wide Approach, 140

slave trade, 7–9, 64, 158, 195

slim disease, 234–35, 239

Southern African Development Commission, 43

stigma, 12; in Ghana, 73, 76; in the Maghreb, 105; in Rwanda, 136; in Tanzania 203, 204, 205; in Uganda 235, 236

structural adjustment programs, 10–11, 196

structural violence, 11

stunting, 210, 211

Tanzania Association of NGOs (TANGO), 213

Tanzania Commission for AIDS, 202

Tebelopele network of VCT centers, 48

tetanus, newborns protected against: in Botswana, *59*; in Ghana, *86*; in the Maghreb, *115*; in Rwanda, *148*; in South Africa, *187*; in Tanzania, *221*; in Uganda, *253*

TF CaRes, Tugela Ferry Care and Research Collaboration, 177

The AIDS Support Organization (TASO), 235, 236

tobacco use, 75

traditional healers or medicine: 12; in Ghana, 72, 74; in Rwanda, 129; in South Africa, 182; in Uganda, 234, 235

traffic accidents. *See* safety, traffic-related

trans-Atlantic slave trade. *See* slave trade

travel clinic, 30–32

Treatment Action Campaign (TAC), 172, 174–75

Truth and Reconciliation Commission, South African, 177

Tuberculosis (TB): in Botswana, 48–50, 51; bovine tuberculosis, 241–42, in Ghana, 77, 79; in Rwanda, 130, 137–38; in South Africa, 156, 157, 168, 175, 176–78, 182; South African mines and, 165–67; in Tanzania, 205–8, 212, 214, 215; TB vaccine trial, 214; in Uganda, 235, 237, 238–39, Ugandan control programme, 233. *See also* HIV/AIDS and tuberculosis

Tulane University, 141

Uganda — Case Western Research Collaboration, 244–45

Uganda Virus Research Institute, 243, 244

UN Millennium Development Goals. *See* Millennium Development Goals

UNAIDS: in Ghana, 78; in Rwanda, 134

UNICEF, 2, 78

University of Botswana, 46, 51

University of California, San Francisco, 213, 245

University of Dar es Salaam's College of Engineering and Technology, 260

University of Ghana, 70, 79

University of Pennsylvania, 50, 51

U.S. Agency for International Development (USAID), 16; in Ghana, 78; in the Maghreb, 109; in Tanzania, 213; in Uganda, 245

violence: in South Africa, 171, 179–81; structural, 11. *See also* violence against women

violence against women: in the Maghreb, 104, 105–8, 120n39; in Rwanda, 134, 135; in South Africa, 180, 181. *See also* domestic violence

visa information, 29–30; for Botswana, 52–53

voluntary counseling and testing (VCT): in Botswana, 48; in Ghana, 76; in Rwanda, 134; in Tanzania, 199, 212; in Uganda, 236, 237

water: bottled, 34; clean, 16, 34; in Tanzania, 211

World Bank, 10, 134

World Health Organization (WHO), 6, 16; in Botswana, 49; in Ghana, 72; guidelines, 49, 239; in the Maghreb, 104; recommendations, 76, 211; in Rwanda, 134; in South Africa, 169, 178; in Tanzania, 211, 212; in Uganda, 243

Women, empowerment of, 74

XDRTB. *See* Extensively Drug-Resistant Tuberculosis

Zoonoses, 241–43

Library of Congress Cataloging-in-Publication Data

Africa: a practical guide for global health workers /
Laurel A. Spielberg and Lisa V. Adams, editors.
    p.; cm.
Includes bibliographical references and index.
ISBN 978-1-58465-976-1 (pbk. : alk. paper)—
ISBN 978-1-61168-018-8 (e-book)
1. World health—Africa. 2. Medical care—
Africa. 3. Altruism—Africa.
I. Spielberg, Laurel A. II. Adams, Lisa V.
[DNLM: 1. Health Status—Africa. 2. Altruism—
Africa. 3. Cultural Characteristics—Africa. 4. Politics—
Africa. 5. World Health—Africa. WA 300 HA1]
RA441.A337   2011
362.1—dc22   2010052990